GRAY'S ANATOMY
COLORING BOOK

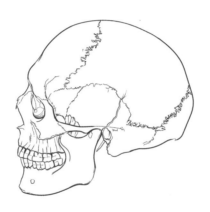

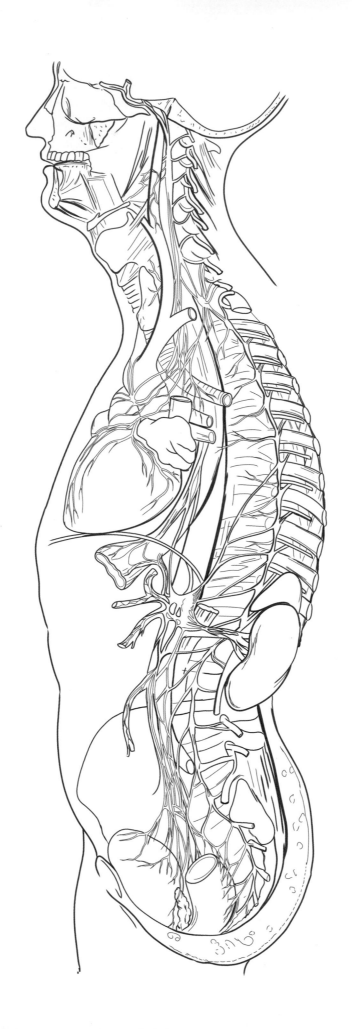

GRAY'S ANATOMY
COLORING BOOK

Images to color from the classic 1860 edition

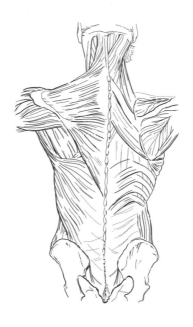

Illustrations by
Chellie Carroll

SIRIUS

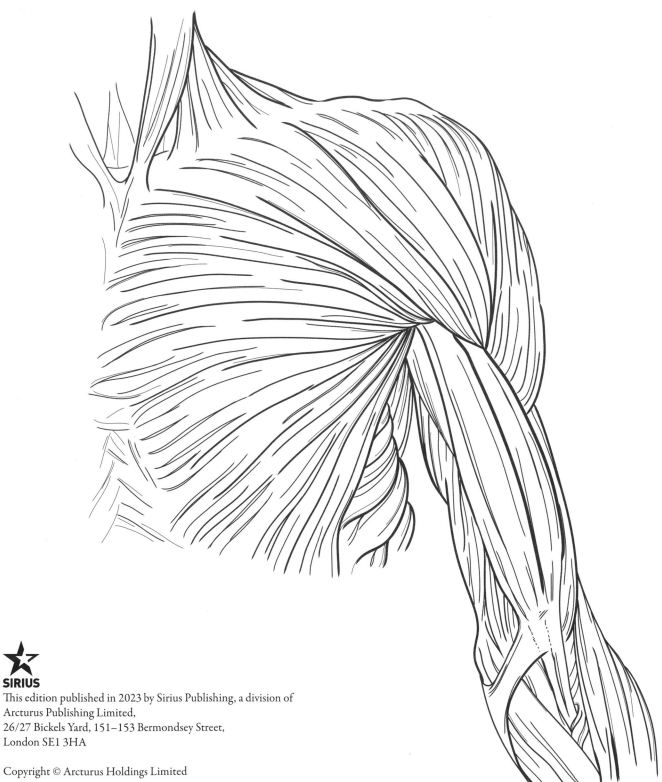

SIRIUS

This edition published in 2023 by Sirius Publishing, a division of
Arcturus Publishing Limited,
26/27 Bickels Yard, 151–153 Bermondsey Street,
London SE1 3HA

ISBN: 978-1-3988-1495-0
CH008735NT
Supplier 29, Date 0223, PI 00000665

Printed in China

INTRODUCTION

When Henry Gray first published his anatomy textbook in 1858, he could not have known that he was about to change the medical world forever. It quickly became a bestseller and it remains today an essential reference guide for every medical professional and student.

Gray's Anatomy owed its success to the intricately detailed and perfectly accurate illustrations provided by Henry Vandyke Carter, which for the first time laid bare every element of the human body, from the bones to the musculature to the essential orders.

In this book you will find recreations of a selection of illustrations from the original textbook, along with Gray's authentic labels and an extract of text about the subject depicted, for you to color in. These images cover the whole range of human anatomy from the bones of the foot to the gray matter that makes up the brain.

Whether you wish to color in the images as accurately as you can or you would prefer to take a more creative approach and turn your imagination loose, you are sure to learn much about the composition of the wonder that is the human body.

In the construction of the human body, it would appear essential, in the first place, to provide some dense and solid texture capable of forming a framework for the support and attachment of the softer parts of the frame, and of forming cavities for the protection of the more important vital organs; and such a structure we find provided in the various bones, which form what is called the skeleton. Bone is one of the hardest structures of the animal body; it possesses also a certain degree of toughness and elasticity. It appears as a pinkish white externally, and deep red within. On examining a section of any bone, it is seen to be composed of two kinds of tissue, one of which is dense and compact in texture, like ivory; the other consisting of slender fibres and lamellae, which join to form a reticular structure; this, from its resemblance to lattice work, is called cancellated.

The compact tissue is always placed on the exterior of a bone; the cancellous tissue is always internal. The relative quantity of these two kinds of tissue varies in different bones, and in different parts of the same bone, as strength or lightness is requisite. Close examination of the compact tissue shows it to be extremely porous, so that the difference in structure between it and the cancellous tissue depends merely upon the different amount of solid matter, and the size and number of the spaces in each; in the compact tissue the cavities being small, and the solid matter between them abundant; whilst in the cancellous tissue the spaces are large, and the solid matter diminished in quantity.

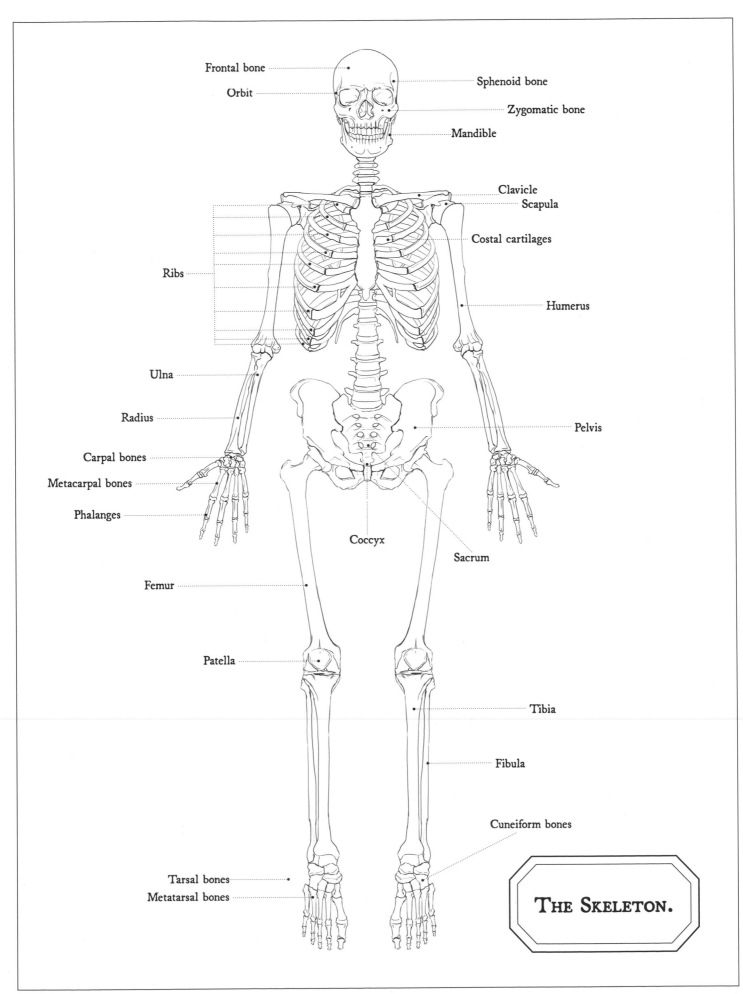

Frontal bone

Orbit

Sphenoid bone

Zygomatic bone

Mandible

Clavicle

Scapula

Costal cartilages

Ribs

Humerus

Ulna

Radius

Pelvis

Carpal bones

Metacarpal bones

Phalanges

Coccyx

Sacrum

Femur

Patella

Tibia

Fibula

Cuneiform bones

Tarsal bones

Metatarsal bones

THE SKELETON.

The anterior region of the skull, which forms the face, is of an oval form, presents an irregular surface, and is excavated for the reception of the two principal organs of sense, the eye and the nose. It is bounded above by the nasal eminences and margins of the orbit; below, by the prominence of the chin; on each side, by the malar bone, and anterior margin of the ramus of the jaw. In the median line are seen from above downwards the nasal eminences, which indicate the situation of the frontal sinuses; diverging outwards from the nasal eminences are the superciliary ridges which support the eyebrows.

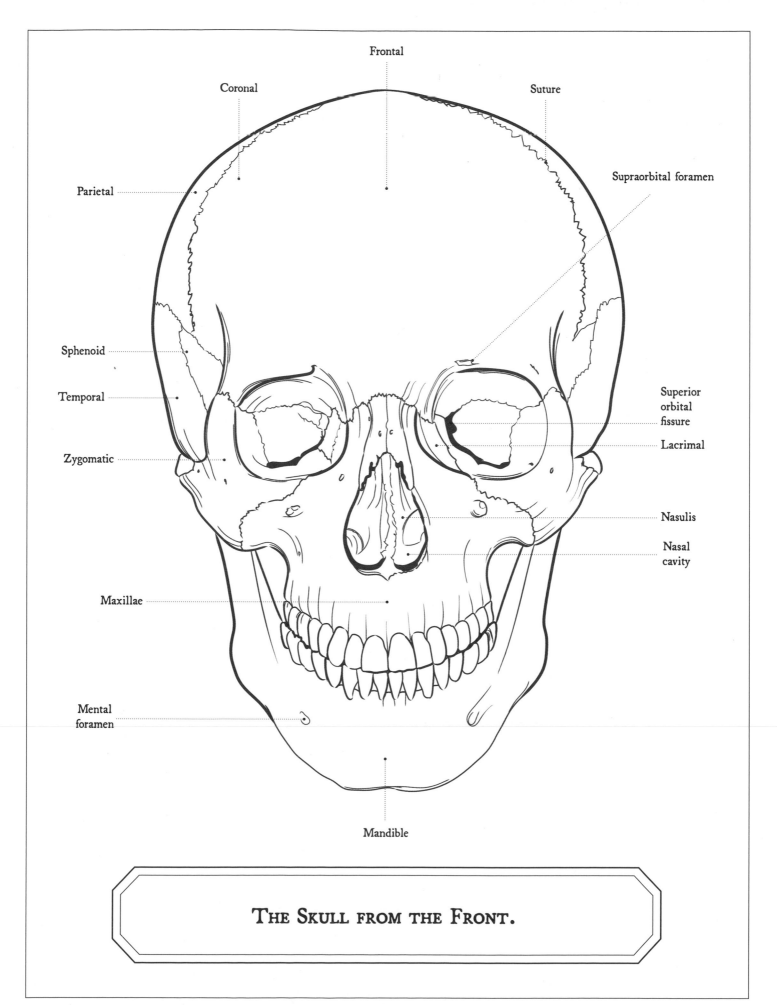

Frontal

Coronal

Suture

Supraorbital foramen

Parietal

Sphenoid

Temporal

Superior
orbital
fissure

Lacrimal

Zygomatic

Nasulis

Nasal
cavity

Maxillae

Mental
foramen

Mandible

THE SKULL FROM THE FRONT.

The lateral region of the skull is somewhat of a triangular
form, its base being formed by a line extending from
the external angular process of the frontal bone along
the temporal ridge backwards to the outer extremity of
the superior curved line of the occiput: and the sides
being formed by two lines, the one drawn downwards and
backwards from the external angular process of the frontal
bone to the angle of the lower jaw, the other from the
angle of the jaw upwards and backwards to the extremity
of the superior curved line. This region is divisible into
three portions: temporal, mastoid and zygomatic.

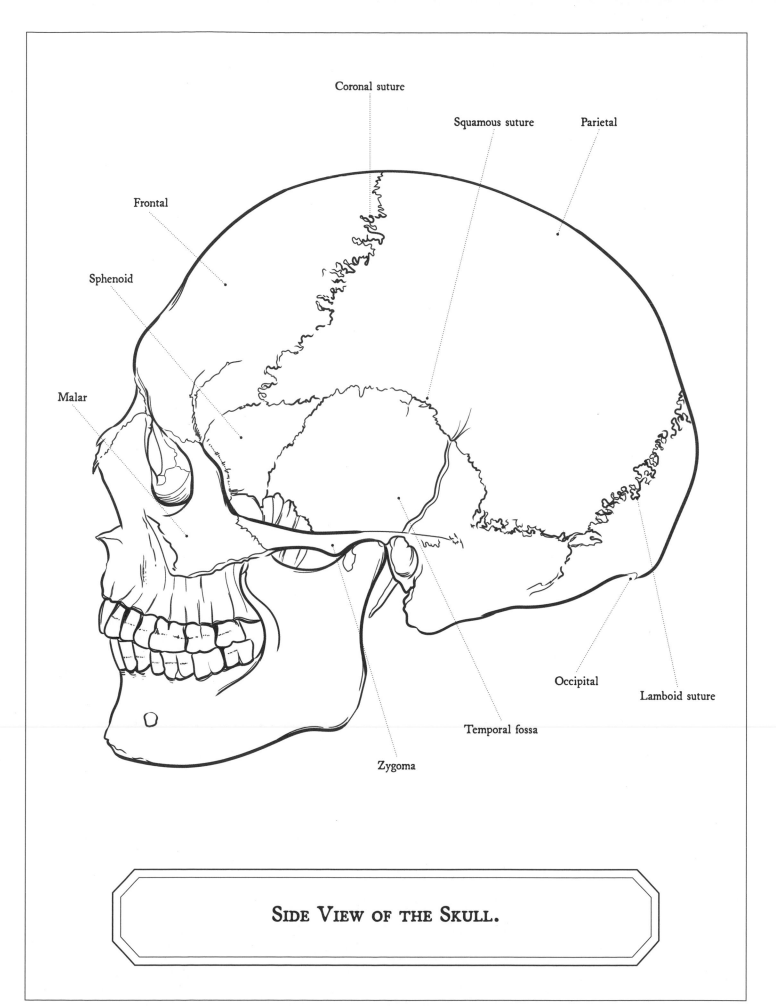

Coronal suture

Squamous suture

Parietal

Frontal

Sphenoid

Malar

Occipital

Lamboid suture

Temporal fossa

Zygoma

SIDE VIEW OF THE SKULL.

The skeleton of the thorax or chest is an osseo-cartilaginous cage, containing and protecting the principal organs of respiration and circulation. It is conical in shape, being narrow above and broad below, flattened from before backward, and longer behind than in front. It is somewhat reniform on transverse section on account of the projection of the vertebral bodies into the cavity.

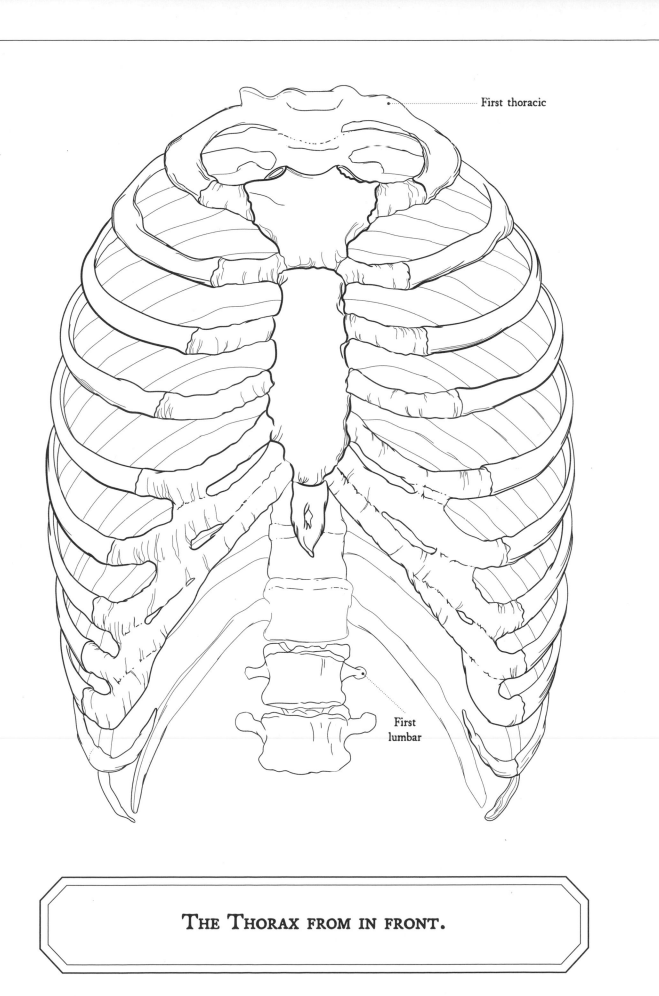

First thoracic

First
lumbar

THE THORAX FROM IN FRONT.

Viewed laterally, the spinal column presents several curves, which correspond to the different regions of the column, and are called cervical, dorsal, lumbar and pelvic. The cervical curve commences at the apex of the odontoid process, and terminates at the middle of the second dorsal vertebra; it is convex in front, but the least marked of all the curves. The dorsal curvature, which is concave forwards, commences at the middle of the second, and terminates at the middle of the twelfth dorsal. Its most prominent point behind corresponds to the body of the seventh or eighth vertebra. The lumbar curve commences at the middle of the last dorsal, and terminates at the sacro-vertebral angle.

It is convex anteriorly; the convexity of the lower three vertebræ being much greater than that of the upper ones. The pelvic curve commences at the sacro-vertebral articulation, and terminates at the point of the coccyx. It is concave posteriorly. The spine has also a slight lateral curvature, the convexity of which is directed toward the right side.

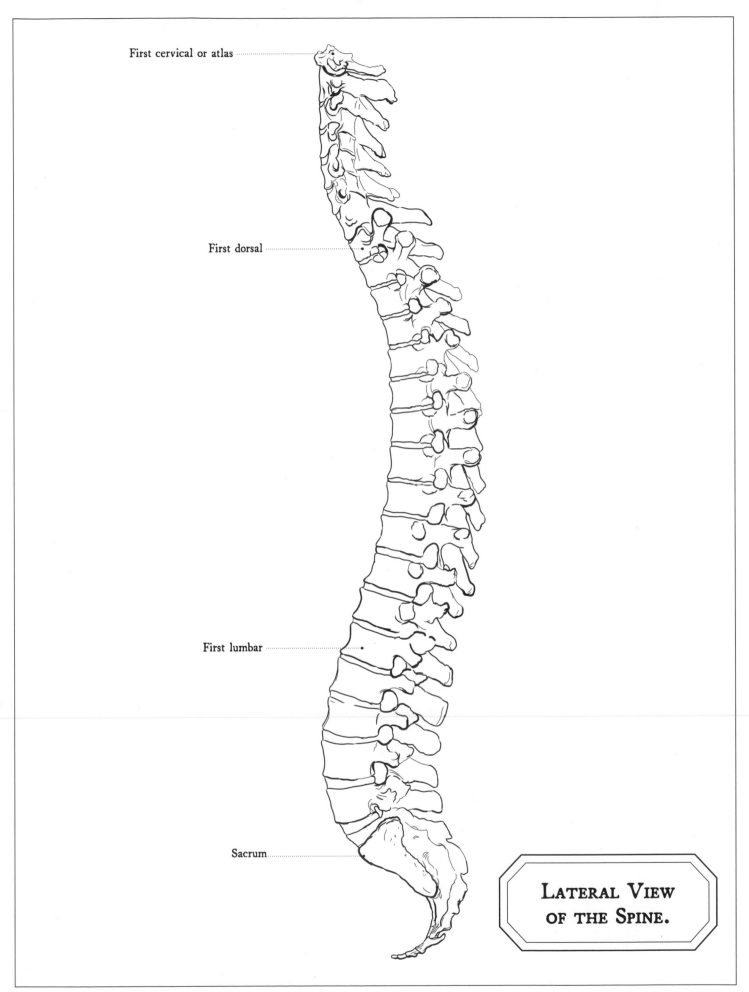

First cervical or atlas

First dorsal

First lumbar

Sacrum

LATERAL VIEW
OF THE SPINE.

The upper extremity consists of the arm, the fore-arm
and the hand. Its continuity with the trunk is established
by means of the shoulder, which is homologous with the
innominate or haunch bone in the lower limb.
The shoulder is placed upon the upper part and side of
the chest, connecting the upper extremity to the trunk;
it consists of two bones, the clavicle and the scapula.
The humerus is the longest and largest bone of the upper
extremity. The ulna, so called from its forming the elbow
(ὠλενη), is a long bone, prismatic in form, placed at the
inner side of the fore-arm, parallel with the radius, being
the largest and longest of the two. The radius (so called
from its fancied resemblance to the spoke of a wheel) is
situated on the outer side of the fore-arm, lying parallel
with the ulna, which exceeds it in length and size. Its
upper end is small, and forms only a small part of the
elbow-joint; but its lower end is large, and forms the
chief part of the wrist. The hand is subdivided into three
segments, the carpus or wrist, the metacarpus or palm
and the phalanges or fingers.

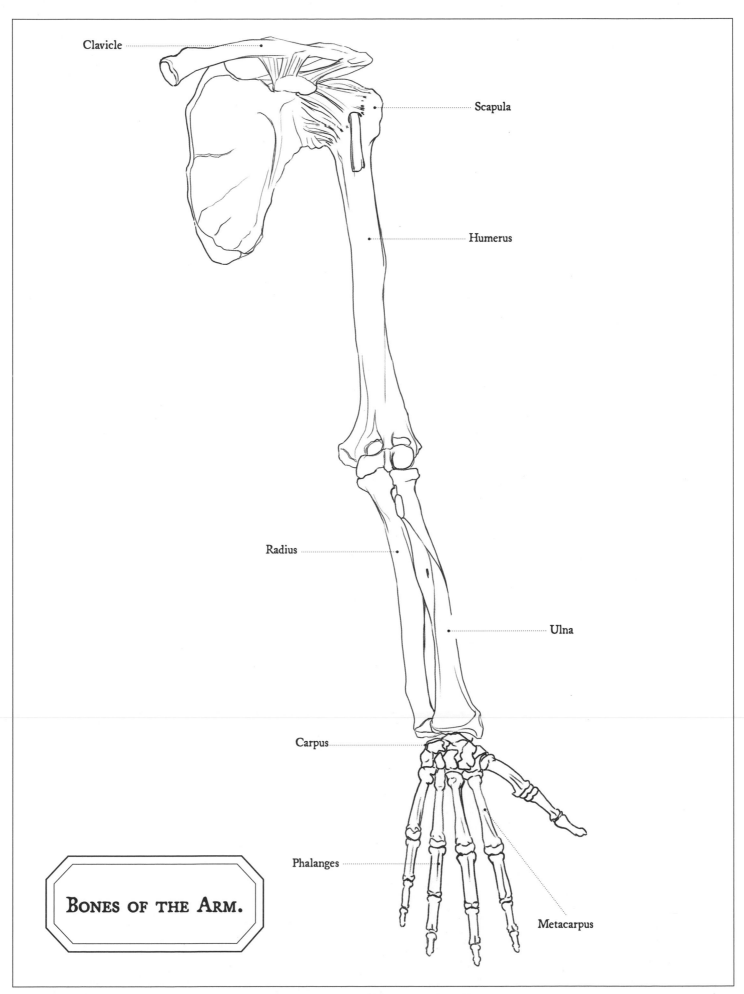

Clavicle

Scapula

Humerus

Radius

Ulna

Carpus

Phalanges

Metacarpus

BONES OF THE ARM.

The hand is subdivided into three segments, the carpus or wrist, the metacarpus or palm and the phalanges or fingers. The bones of the carpus, eight in number, are arranged in two rows. Those of the upper row, enumerated from the radial to the ulnar side, are the scaphoid, semi-lunar, cuneiform and pisiform; those of the lower row, enumerated in the same order, are the trapezium, trapezoid, magnum and unciform.
The metacarpal bones are five in number; they are long cylindrical bones, presenting for examination a shaft and two extremities. The phalanges are the bones of the fingers; they are fourteen in number, three for each finger and two for the thumb. They are long bones, and present for examination a shaft and two extremities.

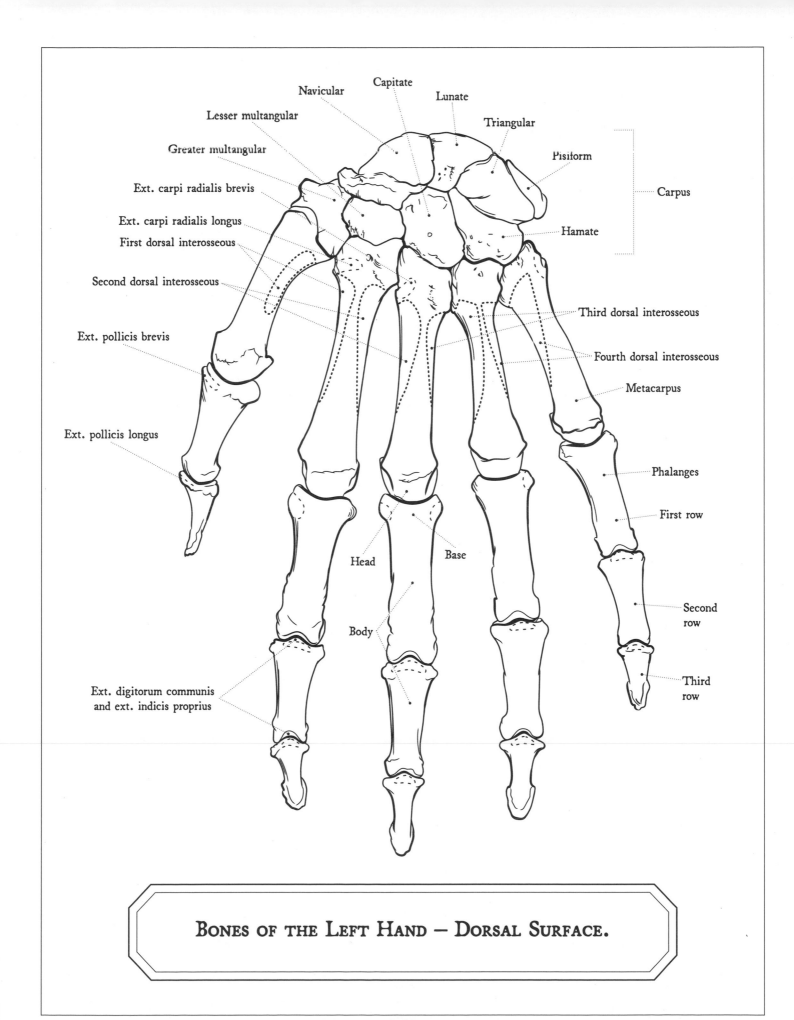

Navicular

Capitate

Lunate

Lesser multangular

Triangular

Greater multangular

Pisiform

Ext. carpi radialis brevis

Carpus

Ext. carpi radialis longus

Hamate

First dorsal interosseous

Second dorsal interosseous

Third dorsal interosseous

Ext. pollicis brevis

Fourth dorsal interosseous

Metacarpus

Ext. pollicis longus

Phalanges

First row

Head

Base

Body

Second row

Third row

Ext. digitorum communis
and ext. indicis proprius

BONES OF THE LEFT HAND – DORSAL SURFACE.

The pelvis, so called from its resemblance to a basin
(πέλυξ), is stronger and more massively constructed
than either of the other osseous cavities; it is a bony
ring, interposed between the lower end of the spine,
which it supports, and the lower extremities, upon which
it rests. It is composed of four bones — the two ossa
innominata, which bound it on either side and in front;
and the sacrum and coccyx, which complete it behind.
In the male, the bones are thicker and stronger, and the
muscular eminences and impressions on their surfaces
more strongly marked. The male pelvis is altogether
more massive; its cavity is deeper and narrower, and
the obturator foramina of larger size. In the female,
the bones are lighter and more expanded, the muscular
impressions on their surfaces are only slightly marked,
and the pelvis generally is less massive in structure.
The iliac fossæ are broad, and the spines of the ilia
widely separated; hence the great prominence of the hips.
The inlet and the outlet are larger; the cavity is more
capacious, and the spines of the ischia project less into it.
The promontory is less projecting, the sacrum wider and
less curved, and the coccyx more moveable.
The arch of the pubes is wider, and its edges more
everted. The tuberosities of the ischia and the acetabula
are wider apart.

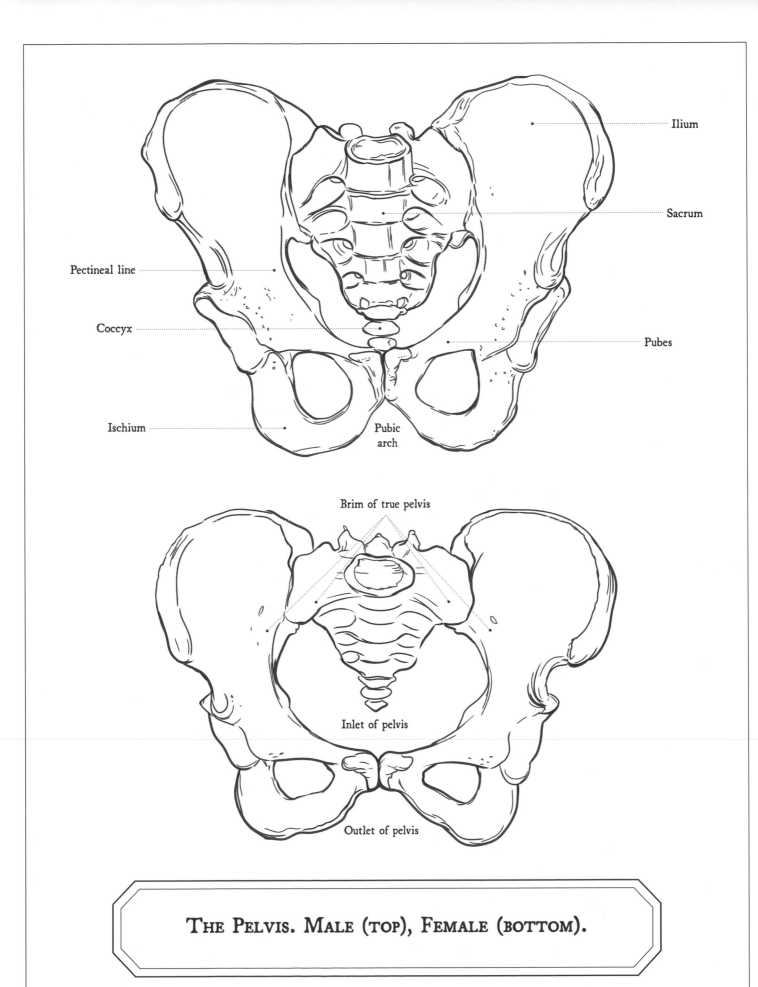

Ilium

Sacrum

Pectineal line

Coccyx

Pubes

Ischium

Pubic arch

Brim of true pelvis

Inlet of pelvis

Outlet of pelvis

THE PELVIS. MALE (TOP), FEMALE (BOTTOM).

This articulation is an enarthrodial, or ball and socket joint, formed by the reception of the head of the femur into the cup-shaped cavity of the acetabulum.

The articulating surfaces are covered with cartilage, that on the head of the femur being thicker at the centre than at the circumference, and covering the entire surface with the exception of a depression just below its centre for the ligamentum teres; that covering the acetabulum is much thinner at the centre than at the circumference, being deficient in the situation of the circular depression at the bottom of this cavity. The ligaments of the joint are:

Capsular. Teres.

Ilio-femoral. Cotyloid.

Transverse.

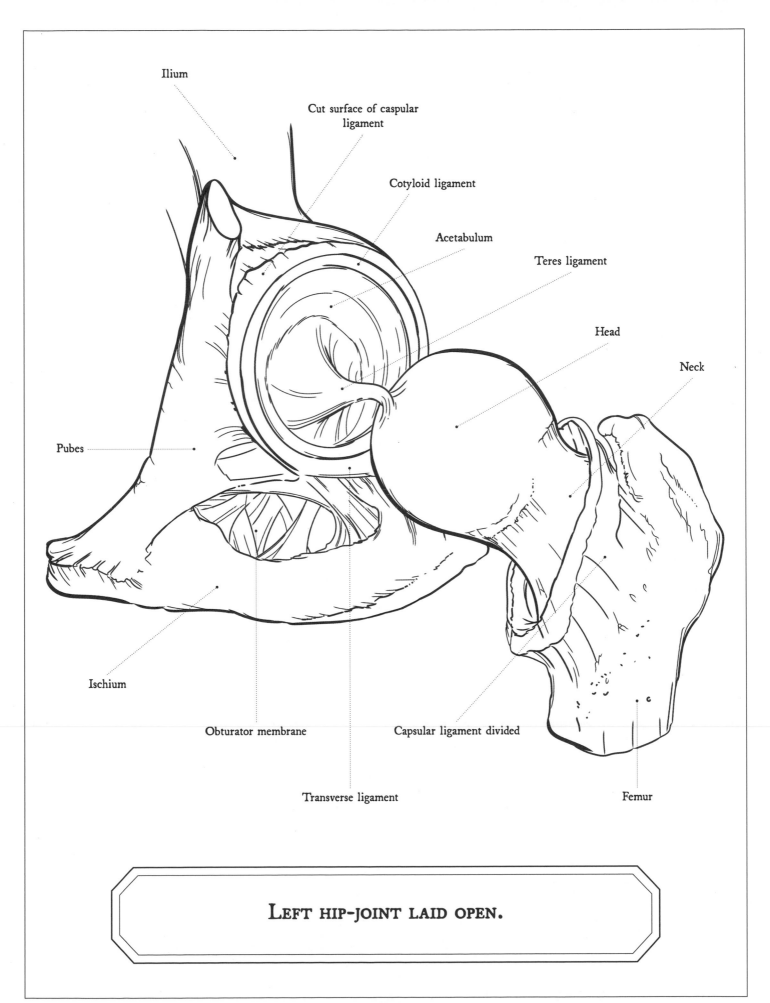

Ilium

Cut surface of caspular
ligament

Cotyloid ligament

Acetabulum

Teres ligament

Head

Neck

Pubes

Ischium

Obturator membrane

Capsular ligament divided

Transverse ligament

Femur

LEFT HIP-JOINT LAID OPEN.

The lower extremity consists of three segments, the thigh, leg and foot, which correspond to the arm, fore-arm and hand in the upper extremity. It is connected to the trunk through the os innominatum, or haunch, which is homologous with the shoulder. The thigh is formed of a single bone, the femur. The femur is the longest, largest and strongest bone in the skeleton, and almost perfectly cylindrical in the greater part of its extent. The leg consists of three bones: the patella, a large sesamoid bone, placed in front of the knee; and the tibia and fibula. The patella is a small, flat, triangular bone, situated at the anterior part of the knee-joint. The tibia (so named from its resemblance to a flute or pipe) is situated at the front and inner side of the leg, and, excepting the femur, is the longest and largest bone in the skeleton. It is prismoid in form, expanded above, where it enters into formation with the knee joint, more slightly enlarged below. The fibula is situated at the outer side of the leg. It is the smaller of the two bones, and, in proportion to its length, the most slender of all the long bones. The foot is the terminal part of the inferior extremity; it serves to support the body in the erect posture, and is an important instrument of locomotion. It consists of three divisions: the tarsus, metatarsus and phalanges.

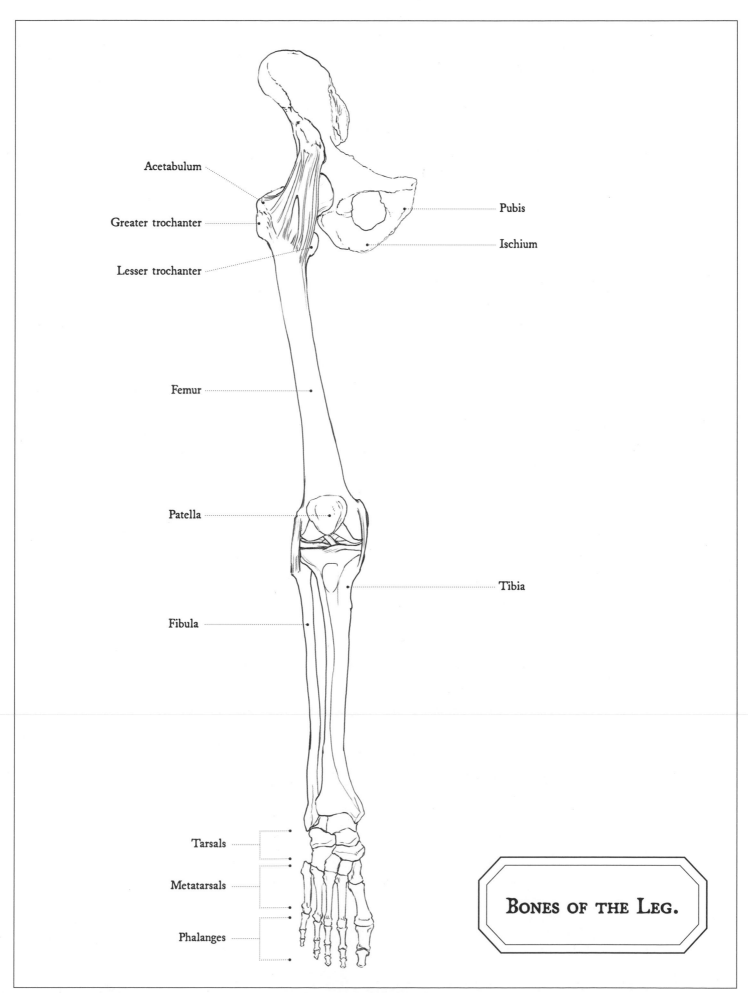

Acetabulum

Greater trochanter

Lesser trochanter

Pubis

Ischium

Femur

Patella

Tibia

Fibula

Tarsals

Metatarsals

Phalanges

BONES OF THE LEG.

The knee is a ginglymoid, or hinge-joint; the bones
entering into its formation are the condyles of the femur
above, the head of the tibia below and the patella in
front. The articular surfaces are covered with cartilage,
and connected together by ligaments, some of which are
placed on the exterior of the joint, whilst others occupy
its interior.

External ligaments. Internal ligaments.
Anterior or ligamentum
patellæ.
Anterior or external crucial.
Posterior or internal crucial.
Posterior or ligamentum posticum
Winslowii.
Two semilunar fibro-cartilages.
Transverse.
Internal lateral. Coronary.
Two external lateral. Ligamentum mucosum.
Capsular. Ligamenta alaria.

The chief movements of this joint are flexion and
extension; but it is also capable of performing some slight
rotatory movement. During flexion, the articular surfaces
of the tibia, covered by their inter-articular cartilages,
glide backwards upon the condyles of the femur, the
lateral, posterior and crucial ligaments are relaxed, the
ligamentum patellæ is put upon the stretch, the patella
filling up the vacuity in front of the joint between the
femur and tibia. In extension, the tibia and inter-articular
cartilages glide forwards upon the femur; all the ligaments
are stretched, with the exception of the ligamentum
patellæ, which is relaxed and admits of considerable
lateral movement. The movement of rotation is permitted
when the knee is semi-flexed, rotation outwards being
most extensive.

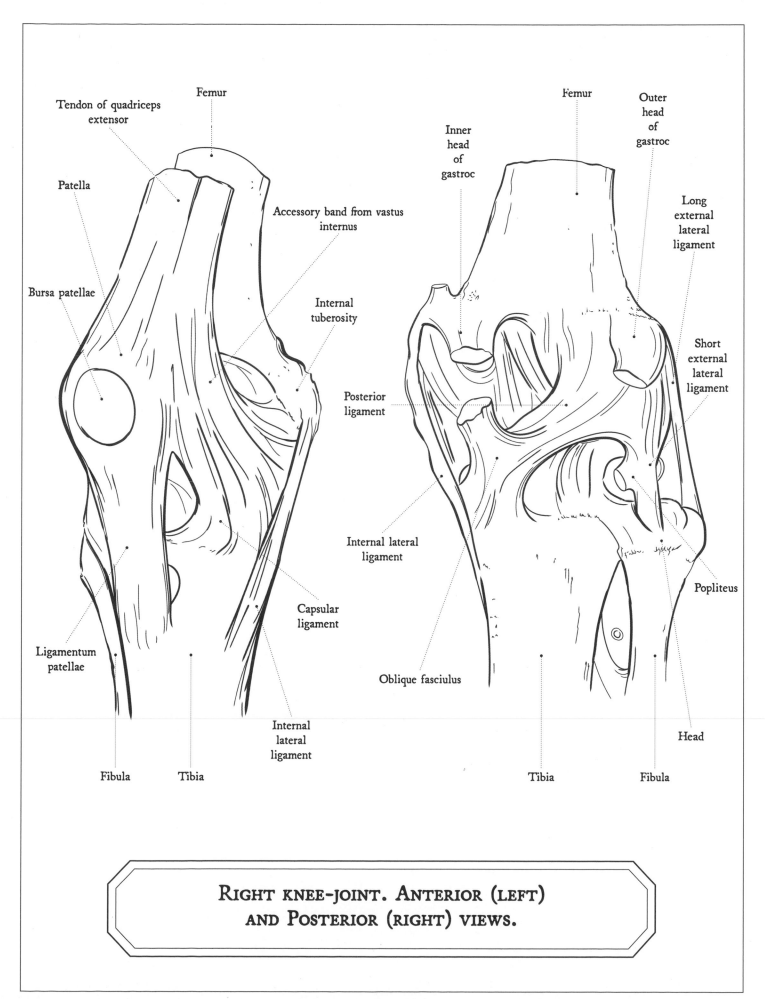

Tendon of quadriceps extensor

Femur

Inner head of gastroc

Femur

Outer head of gastroc

Patella

Accessory band from vastus internus

Long external lateral ligament

Bursa patellae

Internal tuberosity

Short external lateral ligament

Posterior ligament

Internal lateral ligament

Internal lateral ligament

Capsular ligament

Popliteus

Ligamentum patellae

Oblique fasciulus

Head

Fibula

Tibia

Internal lateral ligament

Tibia

Fibula

RIGHT KNEE-JOINT. ANTERIOR (LEFT)
AND POSTERIOR (RIGHT) VIEWS.

The foot is the terminal part of the inferior extremity; it serves to support the body in the erect posture, and is an important instrument of locomotion. It consists of three divisions: the tarsus, metatarsus and phalanges. The bones of the tarsus are seven in number; viz. the calcaneum or os calcis, astragalus, cuboid, scaphoid, internal, middle and external cuneiform bones. The metatarsal bones are five in number; they are long bones, and subdivided into a shaft and two extremities. The phalanges of the foot, both in number and general arrangement, resemble those in the hand, there being two in the great toe and three in each of the other toes.

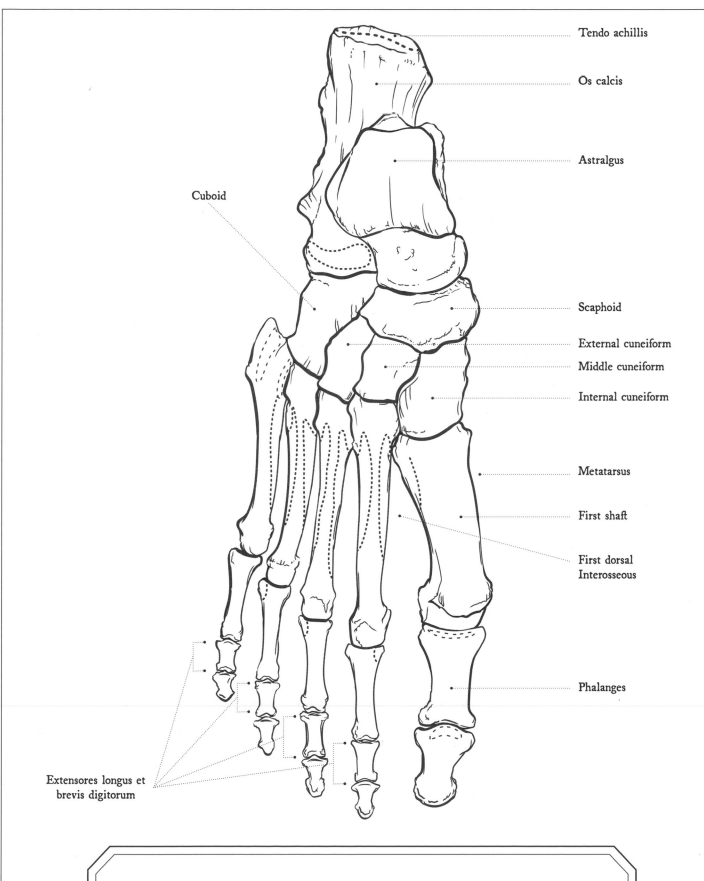

Tendo achillis

Os calcis

Astralgus

Cuboid

Scaphoid

External cuneiform

Middle cuneiform

Internal cuneiform

Metatarsus

First shaft

First dorsal
Interosseous

Phalanges

Extensores longus et
brevis digitorum

BONES OF THE RIGHT FOOT. DORSAL SURFACE.

The muscles are the active organs of locomotion. They are formed of bundles of reddish fibres, consisting chemically of fibrine and endowed with the property of contractility. Two kinds of muscular tissue are found in the animal body, viz. that of voluntary or animal life, and that of involuntary or organic life. The muscles of animal life (striped muscles) are composed of bundles of fibres enclosed in a delicate web of areolar tissue. Each bundle consists of numerous smaller ones, enclosed in a similar fibro-areolar covering, and these again of primitive fasciculi.

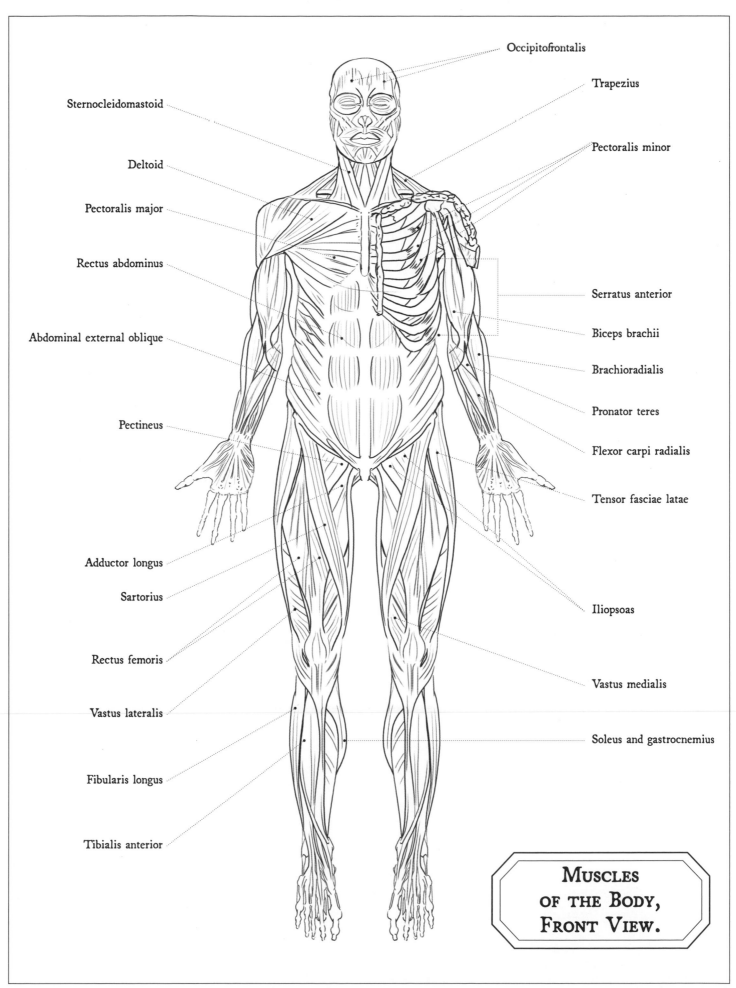

Occipitofrontalis

Trapezius

Sternocleidomastoid

Pectoralis minor

Deltoid

Pectoralis major

Rectus abdominus

Serratus anterior

Abdominal external oblique

Biceps brachii

Brachioradialis

Pronator teres

Pectineus

Flexor carpi radialis

Tensor fasciae latae

Adductor longus

Sartorius

Rectus femoris

Iliopsoas

Vastus lateralis

Vastus medialis

Soleus and gastrocnemius

Fibularis longus

Tibialis anterior

MUSCLES
OF THE BODY,
FRONT VIEW.

The muscles of the trunk may be subdivided
into four groups:

1. Muscles of the back.
2. Muscles of the abdomen.
3. Muscles of the thorax.
4. Muscles of the perinæum.

The muscles of organic life (unstriped muscles) consist
of flattened bands, or of elongated, spindle-shaped
fibres, flattened, of a pale appearance, homogeneous in
texture, having a finely mottled aspect. Blood-vessels are
distributed in considerable abundance to the muscular
tissue. Each muscle is invested externally by a thin
cellular layer, forming what is called its sheath, which
not only covers its outer surface, but penetrates into its
interior in the intervals between the fasciculi, surrounding
these and serving as a bond of connection between
them. The muscles are connected with the bones,
cartilages, ligaments and skin, either directly or through
the intervention of fibrous structures, called tendons or
aponeuroses. The muscles vary considerably in their form.
In the limbs, they are of considerable length, especially
the more superficial ones, the deep ones being generally
broad; they surround the bones, and form an important
protection to the various joints. In the trunk, they are
broad, flattened and expanded, forming the parieties of the
cavities which they enclose.

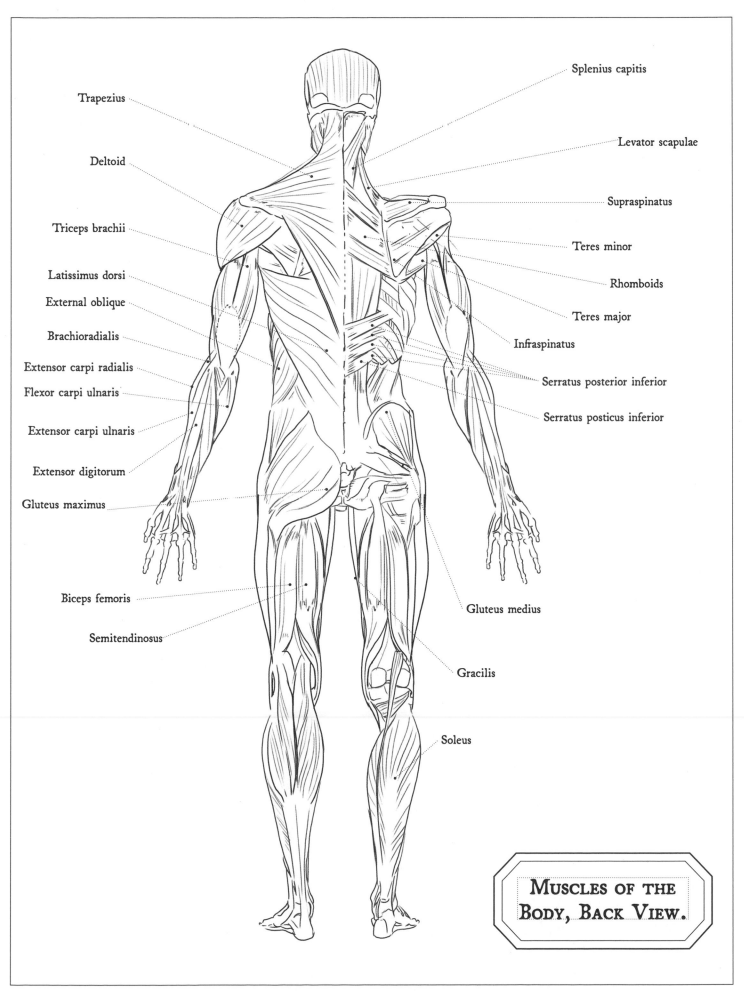

Trapezius

Deltoid

Triceps brachii

Latissimus dorsi

External oblique

Brachioradialis

Extensor carpi radialis

Flexor carpi ulnaris

Extensor carpi ulnaris

Extensor digitorum

Gluteus maximus

Biceps femoris

Semitendinosus

Splenius capitis

Levator scapulae

Supraspinatus

Teres minor

Rhomboids

Teres major

Infraspinatus

Serratus posterior inferior

Serratus posticus inferior

Gluteus medius

Gracilis

Soleus

MUSCLES OF THE
BODY, BACK VIEW.

The muscles of the head and face consist of ten groups,
arranged according to the region in which they are situated.

1. Cranial region.
2. Auricular region.
3. Palpebral region.
4. Orbital region.
5. Nasal region.

6. Superior maxillary region.
7. Inferior maxillary region.
8. Inter-maxillary region.
9. Temporo-maxillary region.
10. Pterygo-maxillary region.

The muscles of the neck may be arranged into groups,
corresponding with the region in which they are situated.
These groups are nine in number:—

1. Superficial region.
2. Depressors of the os hyoides and larynx.
3. Elevators of the os hyoides and larynx.
4. Muscles of the tongue.
5. Muscles of the pharynx.

6. Muscles of the soft palate.
7. Muscles of the anterior vertebral region.
8. Muscles of the lateral vertebral region.
9. Muscles of the larynx.

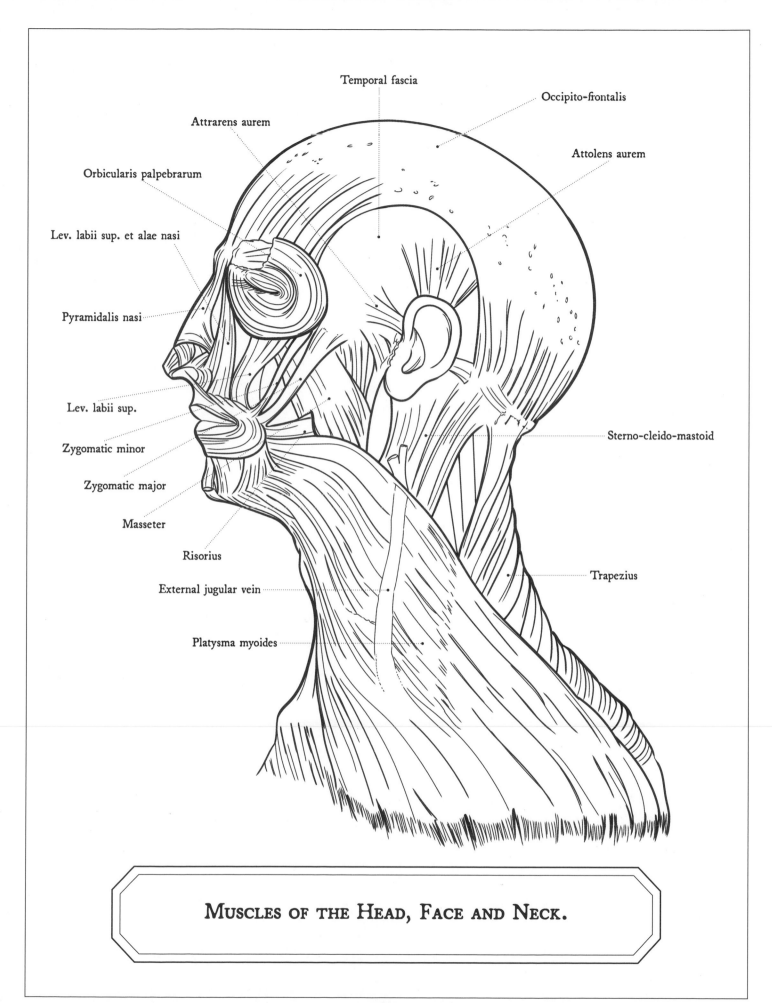

Temporal fascia

Occipito-frontalis

Attrarens aurem

Attolens aurem

Orbicularis palpebrarum

Lev. labii sup. et alae nasi

Pyramidalis nasi

Lev. labii sup.

Zygomatic minor

Zygomatic major

Masseter

Risorius

External jugular vein

Platysma myoides

Sterno-cleido-mastoid

Trapezius

MUSCLES OF THE HEAD, FACE AND NECK.

The muscles of the neck may be arranged into groups, corresponding with the region in which they are situated. These groups are nine in number:—

1. Superficial region.
2. Depressors of the os hyoides and larynx.
3. Elevators of the os hyoides and larynx.
4. Muscles of the tongue.
5. Muscles of the pharynx.
6. Muscles of the soft palate.
7. Muscles of the anterior vertebral region.
8. Muscles of the lateral vertebral region.
9. Muscles of the larynx.

The sterno-cleido-mastoid is a large thick muscle, which passes obliquely across the side of the neck, being enclosed between the two layers of the deep cervical fascia. The supra-hyoid region muscles (consisting of the digastric, stylo-hyoid, mylo-hyoid and genio-hyoid muscles) raise the hyoid base, and with it the base of the tongue or they depress the lower jaw.

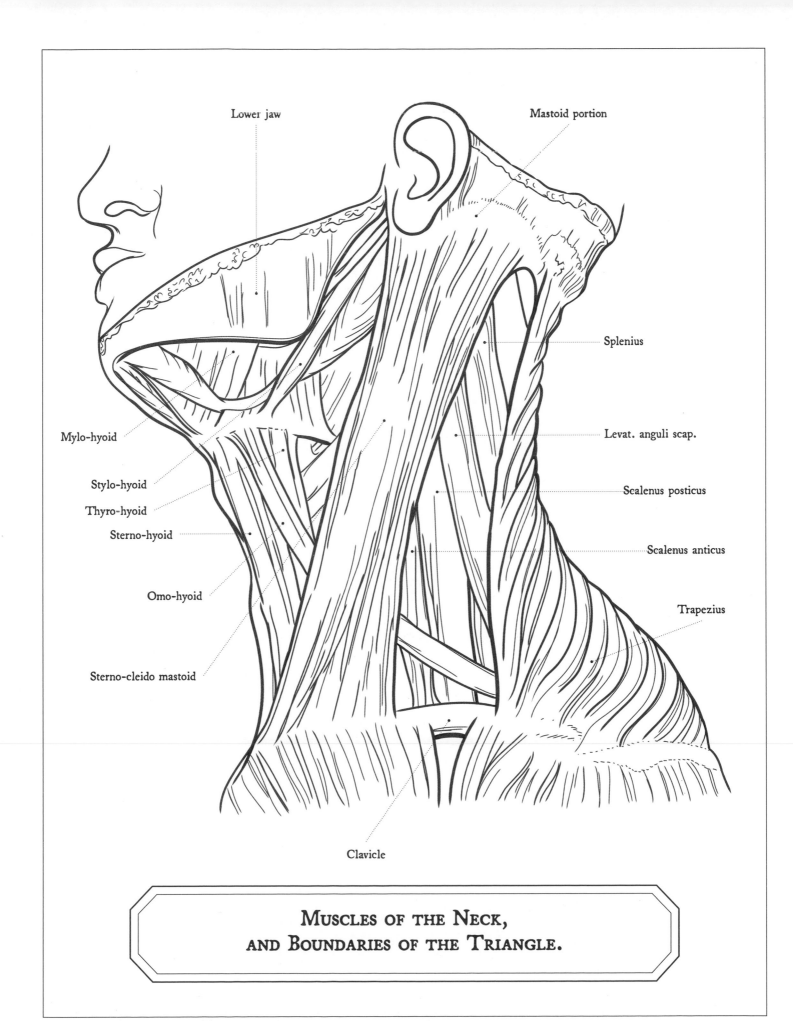

Lower jaw

Mastoid portion

Splenius

Mylo-hyoid

Levat. anguli scap.

Stylo-hyoid

Thyro-hyoid

Scalenus posticus

Sterno-hyoid

Scalenus anticus

Omo-hyoid

Trapezius

Sterno-cleido mastoid

Clavicle

MUSCLES OF THE NECK, AND BOUNDARIES OF THE TRIANGLE.

The pectoralis major is a broad, thick, triangular muscle, situated at the upper and fore part of the chest.

The deltoid is a large, thick triangular muscle, which forms the convexity of the shoulder. The deltoid raises the arm directly from the side, so as to bring it at right angles with the trunk. Its anterior fibres, assisted by the pectoralis major, draw the arm forwards; and its posterior fibres, aided by the teres major and latissimus dorsi, draw it backwards. If the arm has been raised by the deltoid, the pectoralis major will, conjointly with the latissimus dorsi and teres major, depress it to the side of the chest; and if acting singly, it will draw the arm across the front of the chest.

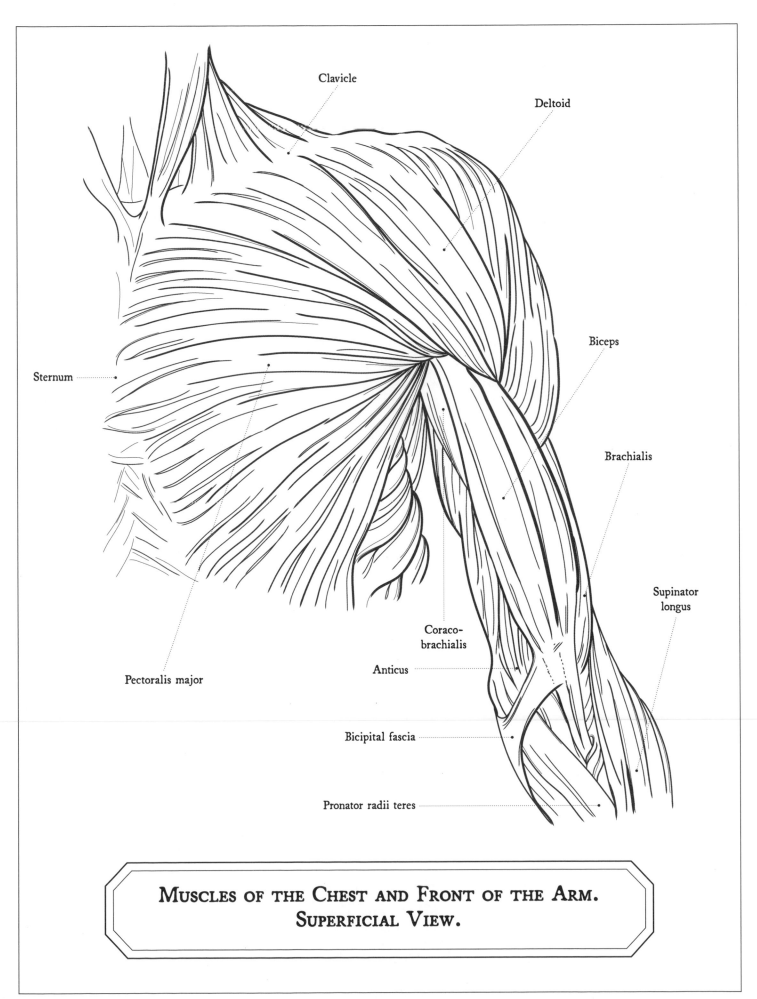

Clavicle

Deltoid

Biceps

Brachialis

Sternum

Supinator
longus

Coraco-
brachialis

Anticus

Pectoralis major

Bicipital fascia

Pronator radii teres

MUSCLES OF THE CHEST AND FRONT OF THE ARM.
SUPERFICIAL VIEW.

The triceps is situated on the back of the arm, extending the entire length of the posterior surface of the humerus. It is of large size, and divided above into three parts; hence the name of the muscle. These three portions have been named the middle or long head, the external and the internal head. The triceps is the great extensor muscle of the fore-arm; when the fore-arm is flexed, serving to draw it into a right line with the arm. It is the direct antagonist of the biceps and brachialis anticus. When the arm is extended, the long head of the muscle may assist the teres major and latissimus dorsi in drawing the humerus backwards. The long head of the triceps protects the under part of the shoulder-joint, and prevents displacement of the head of the humerus downwards and backwards.

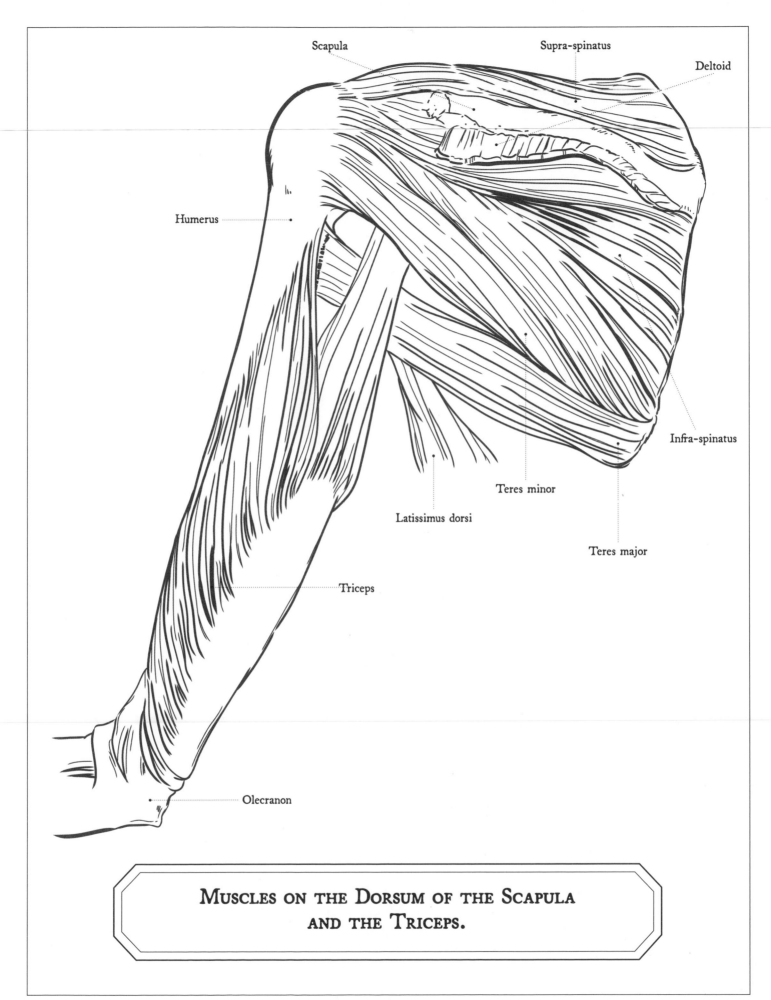

Scapula

Supra-spinatus

Deltoid

Humerus

Infra-spinatus

Teres minor

Latissimus dorsi

Teres major

Triceps

Olecranon

**MUSCLES ON THE DORSUM OF THE SCAPULA
AND THE TRICEPS.**

Muscles of the back. On the left side is exposed the first layer, on the right side, the second layer and part of the third. The trapezius is a broad, flat, triangular muscle placed immediately beneath the skin, and covering the upper and back part of the neck and shoulders. The latissimus dorsi is a broad flat muscle, which covers the lumbar and lower half of the dorsal regions. If the head is fixed, the upper part of the trapezius will elevate the point of the shoulder, as in supporting weights; when the middle and lower fibres are brought into action, partial rotation of the scapula upon the side of the chest is produced. If the shoulders are fixed, the trapezii will draw the head directly backwards, or if only one acts, to the corresponding side. The latissimus dorsi draws the humerus backwards and downwards and rotates it inwards. If the arm is fixed, it may raise the lower ribs and assist in forcible inspiration, or if both arms are fixed, it may assist with the abdominal and pectoral muscles in drawing the whole trunk forwards. The rhomboid muscles carry the inferior angle backwards and upwards, thus producing a slight rotation of the scapula upon the side of the chest.

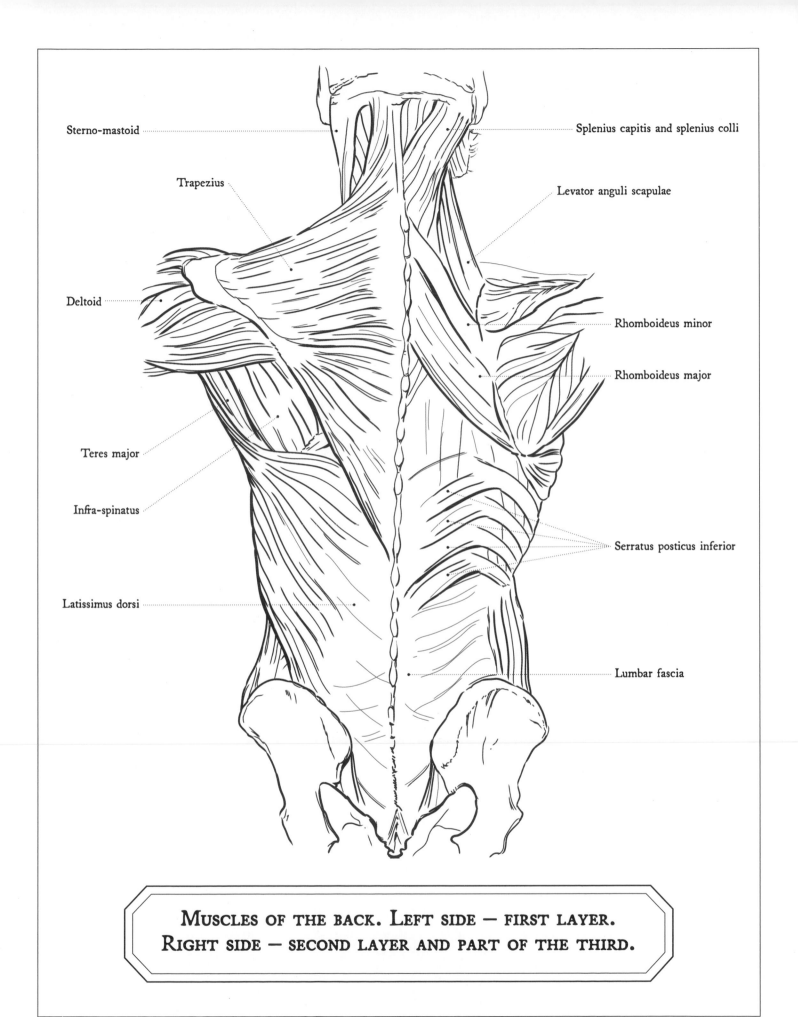

Sterno-mastoid

Trapezius

Deltoid

Teres major

Infra-spinatus

Latissimus dorsi

Splenius capitis and splenius colli

Levator anguli scapulae

Rhomboideus minor

Rhomboideus major

Serratus posticus inferior

Lumbar fascia

MUSCLES OF THE BACK. LEFT SIDE — FIRST LAYER.
RIGHT SIDE — SECOND LAYER AND PART OF THE THIRD.

The external oblique muscle, so called from the direction of its fibres, is situated on the side and fore part of the abdomen; being the largest and the most superficial of the three flat muscles in this region. It is broad, thin, irregularly quadrilateral in form, its muscular portion occupying the side, its aponeurosis the anterior wall of that cavity. It arises, by eight fleshy digitations, from the external surface and lower borders of the eight inferior ribs; these digitations are arranged in an oblique line running downwards and backwards; the upper ones being attached close to the cartilages of the corresponding ribs; the lowest, to the apex of the cartilage of the last rib; the intermediate ones, to the ribs at some distance from their cartilages. The five superior serrations increase in size from above downwards, and are received between corresponding processes of the serratus magnus; the three lower ones diminish in size from above downwards, receiving between them corresponding processes from the latissimus dorsi.

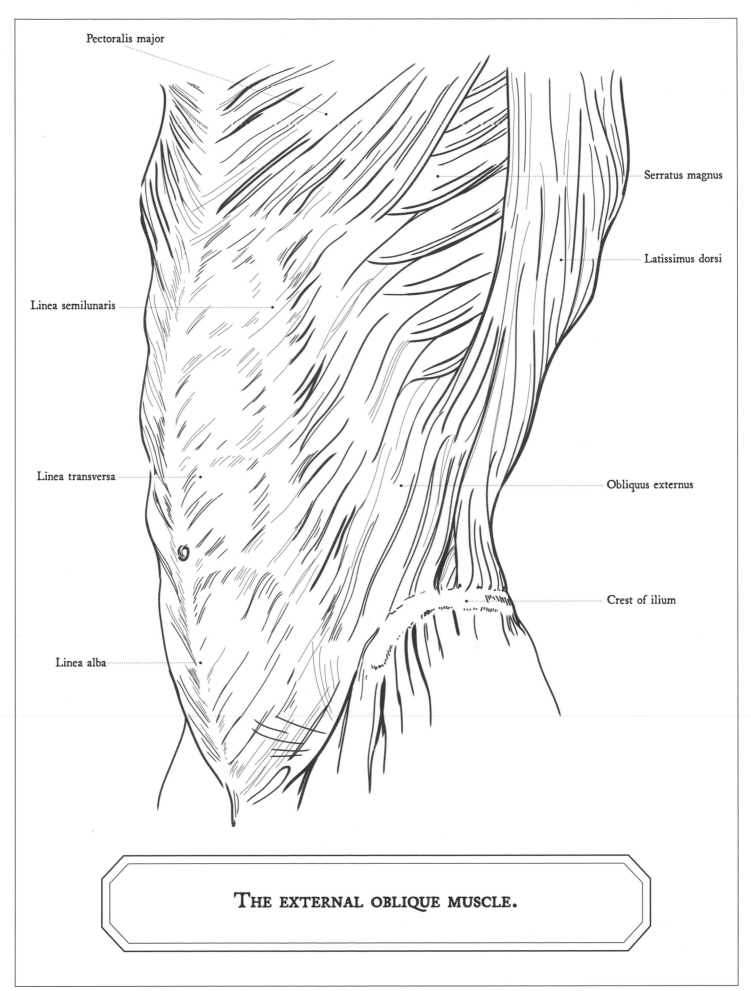

Pectoralis major

Serratus magnus

Latissimus dorsi

Linea semilunaris

Linea transversa

Obliquus externus

Crest of ilium

Linea alba

THE EXTERNAL OBLIQUE MUSCLE.

The transversalis muscle, so called from the direction
of its fibres, is the most internal flat muscle of the
abdomen, being placed immediately beneath the internal
oblique. The rectus abdominis is a long, flat muscle,
which extends along the whole length of the front of the
abdomen, being separated from its fellow of the opposite
side by the linea alba. The rectus muscle is traversed
by a series of tendinous intersections, which vary from
two to five in number, and have received the name lineæ
transversæ. The rectus is enclosed in a sheath, formed by
the aponeuroses of the oblique and transversalis muscles.
The pyramidalis is a small muscle, triangular in form,
placed at the lower part of the abdomen, in front of the
rectus, and contained in the same sheath with
that muscle.

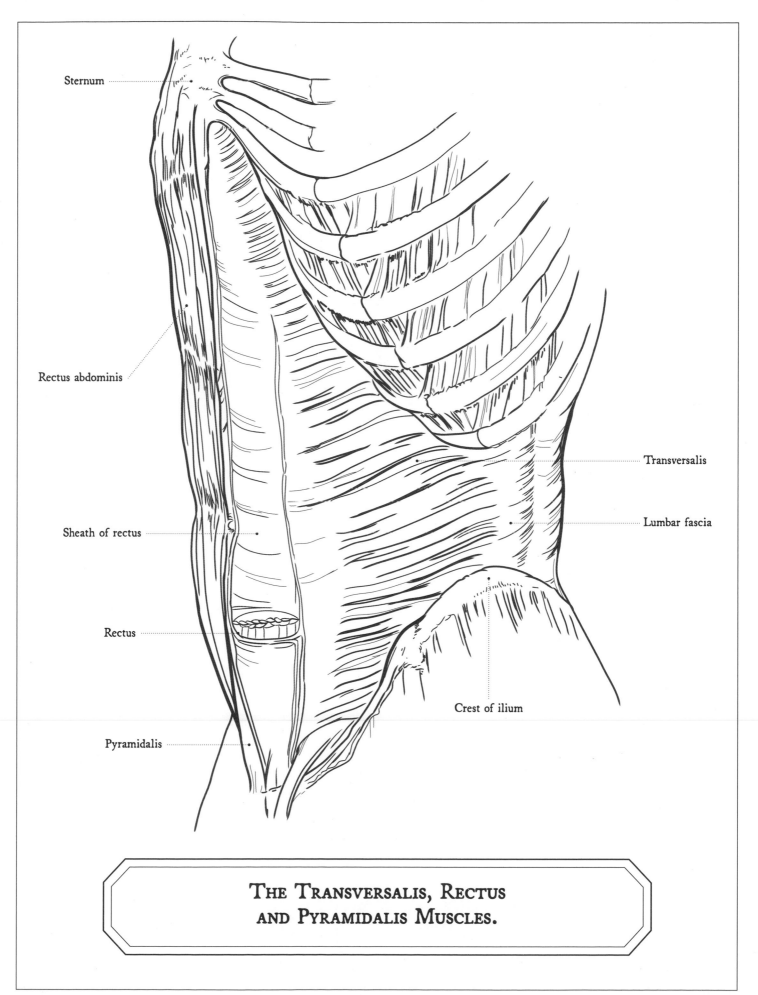

Sternum

Rectus abdominis

Sheath of rectus

Rectus

Pyramidalis

Transversalis

Lumbar fascia

Crest of ilium

THE TRANSVERSALIS, RECTUS AND PYRAMIDALIS MUSCLES.

The muscles of the fore-arm may be subdivided into groups: the inner and anterior aspect, comprising the flexor and pronator muscles; the outer side of the fore-arm; and the posterior aspect. The two latter groups include all the extensor and supinator muscles. The muscles of the radial and posterior brachial regions, which comprise all the extensor and supinator muscles, act upon the fore-arm, wrist and hand; they are the direct antagonists of the pronator and flexor muscles. The anconeus assists the triceps in extending the fore-arm. The supinator longus and brevis are the supinators of the fore-arm and hand; the former muscle more especially acting as a supinator when the limb is pronated. When supination has been produced, the supinator longus, if still continuing to act, flexes the fore-arm.

The extensor carpi radialis longior and brevior, and extensor carpi ulnaris muscles, are the extensors of the wrist; continuing their action, they serve to extend the fore-arm upon the arm; they are the direct antagonists of the flexor carpi radialis and ulnaris.

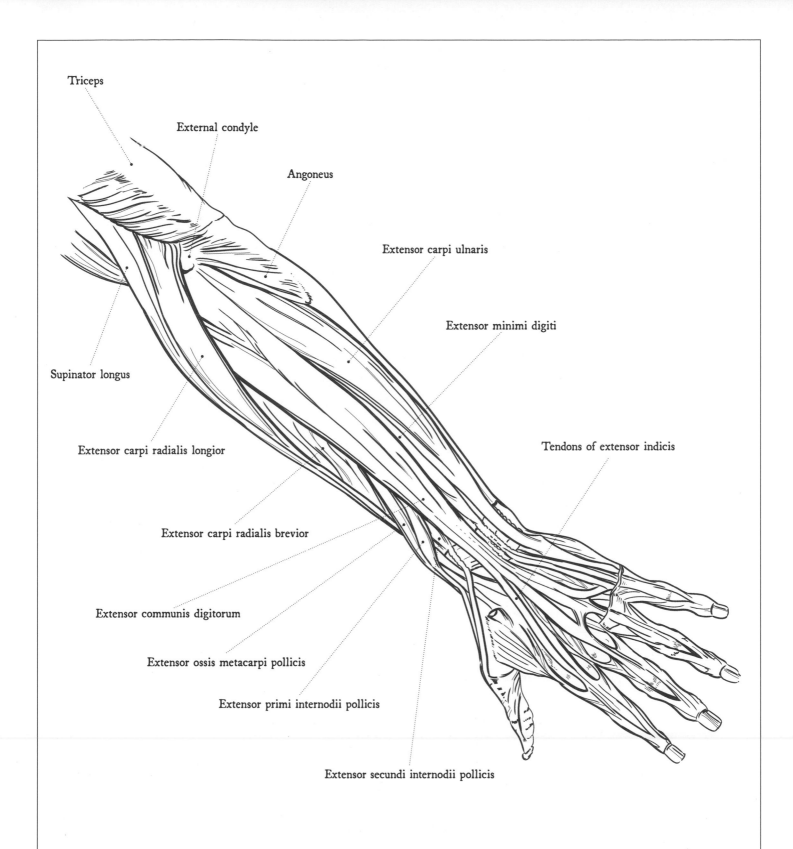

Triceps

External condyle

Angoneus

Extensor carpi ulnaris

Extensor minimi digiti

Supinator longus

Tendons of extensor indicis

Extensor carpi radialis longior

Extensor carpi radialis brevior

Extensor communis digitorum

Extensor ossis metacarpi pollicis

Extensor primi internodii pollicis

Extensor secundi internodii pollicis

POSTERIOR SURFACE OF FORE-ARM.
SUPERFICIAL MUSCLES.

The psoas and iliacus muscles, acting from above, flex the
thigh upon the pelvis, and, at the same time, rotate the
femur outwards, from the obliquity of their insertion into
the inner and back part of that bone. Acting from below,
the femur being fixed, the muscles of both sides bend the
lumbar portion of the spine and pelvis forwards.
They also serve to maintain the erect position, by
supporting the spine and pelvis upon the femur, and
assist in raising the trunk when the body is in the
recumbent posture.

The tensor vaginæ femoris is a tensor of the fascia
lata; continuing its action, the oblique direction of its
fibres enables it to rotate the thigh inwards. In the
erect posture, acting from below, it will serve to steady
the pelvis upon the head of the femur. The sartorius
flexes the leg upon the thigh, and, continuing to act,
the thigh upon the pelvis, at the same time drawing
the limb inwards, so as to cross one leg over the other.
Taking its fixed point from the leg, it flexes the pelvis
upon the thigh, and, if one muscle acts, assists in
rotating it. The quadriceps extensor extends the leg
upon the thigh. Taking its fixed point from the leg, as in
standing, this muscle will act upon the femur, supporting
it perpendicularly upon the head of the tibia, thus
maintaining the entire weight of the body.
The rectus muscle assists the psoas and iliacus, in
supporting the pelvis and trunk upon the femur, or in
bending it forwards.

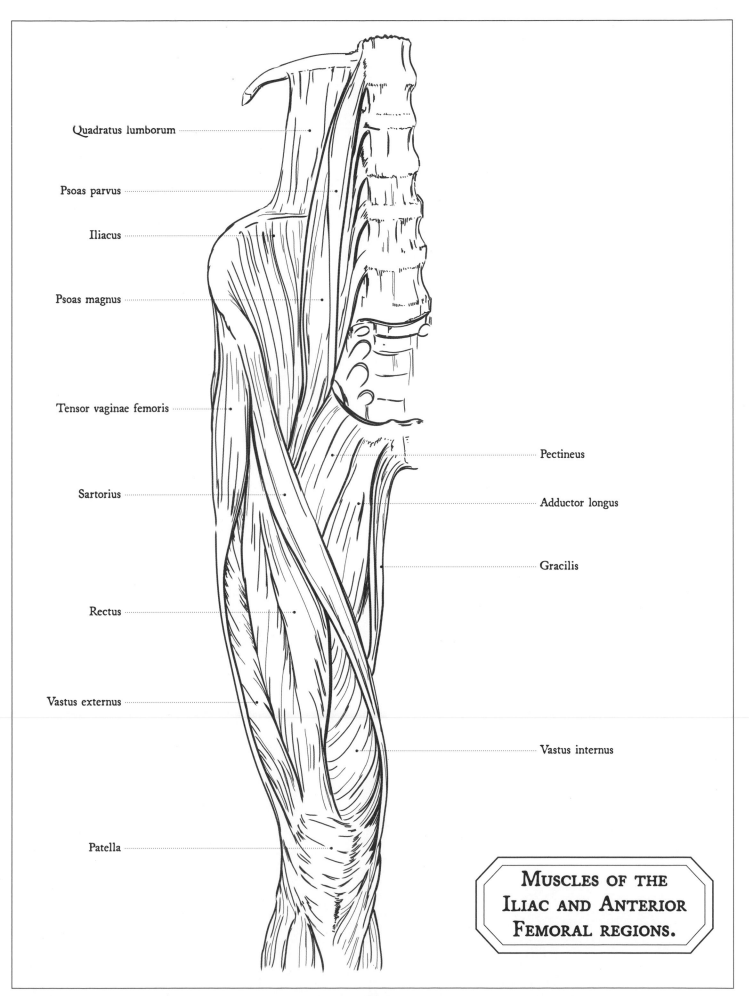

Quadratus lumborum

Psoas parvus

Iliacus

Psoas magnus

Tensor vaginae femoris

Sartorius

Rectus

Vastus externus

Patella

Pectineus

Adductor longus

Gracilis

Vastus internus

MUSCLES OF THE
ILIAC AND ANTERIOR
FEMORAL REGIONS.

The leg muscles may be subdivided into three groups: those on the anterior, those on the posterior and those on the outer side. The tibialis anticus is situated on the outer side of the tibia. The extensor longus digitorum is an elongated, flattened, semi-penniform muscle, situated the most externally of all the muscles on the fore-part of the leg. The tibialis anticus and peroneus tertius are the direct flexors of the tarsus upon the leg; the former raises the inner border of the foot, and the latter will draw the outer border of the foot upwards and the sole outwards.

The extensor longus digitorum and extensor proprius pollicis extend the phallanges of the toes, and continuing their action, flex the tarsus upon the leg.

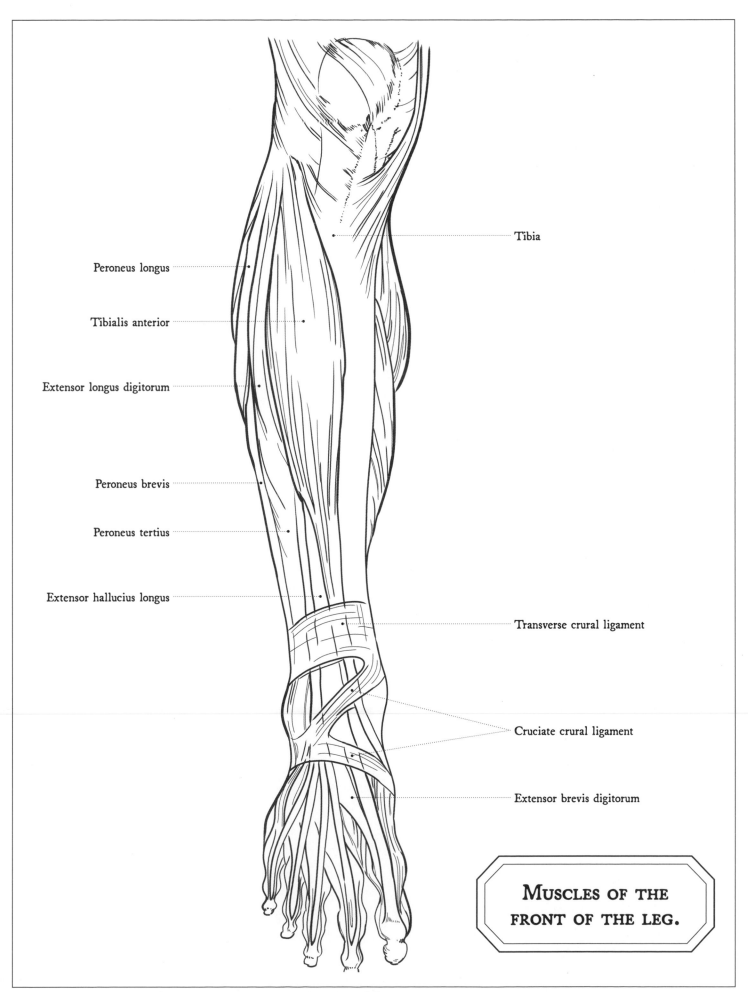

Peroneus longus

Tibialis anterior

Extensor longus digitorum

Peroneus brevis

Peroneus tertius

Extensor hallucius longus

Tibia

Transverse crural ligament

Cruciate crural ligament

Extensor brevis digitorum

MUSCLES OF THE FRONT OF THE LEG.

The muscles in this region of the leg are subdivided into two layers, superficial and deep. The superficial layer constitutes a powerful muscular mass, forming what is called the calf. The Gastrocnemius is the most superficial muscle, and forms the greater part of the calf. The Soleus is a broad flat muscle, situated immediately beneath the preceding. The tendo Achillis is the thickest and strongest tendon in the body. The muscles of the calf possess considerable power, and are constantly called into use in standing, walking, dancing, and leaping; hence the large size they usually present.

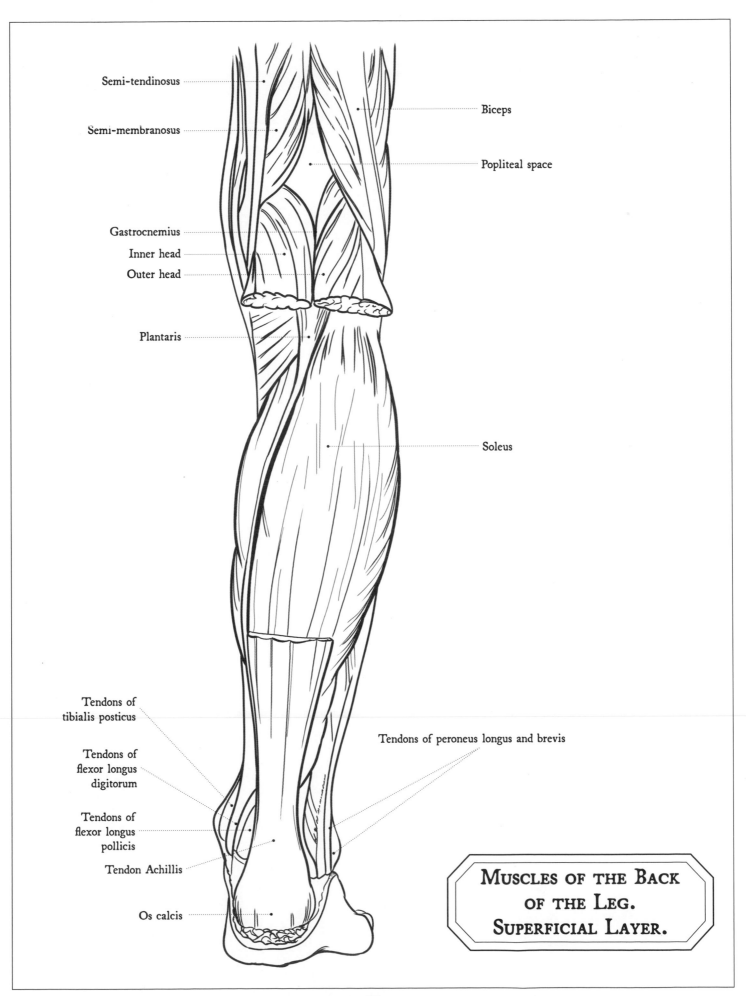

Semi-tendinosus

Semi-membranosus

Biceps

Popliteal space

Gastrocnemius

Inner head

Outer head

Plantaris

Soleus

Tendons of
tibialis posticus

Tendons of
flexor longus
digitorum

Tendons of peroneus longus and brevis

Tendons of
flexor longus
pollicis

Tendon Achillis

MUSCLES OF THE BACK
OF THE LEG.
SUPERFICIAL LAYER.

Os calcis

The apparatus for the digestion of the food consists of the alimentary canal, and of certain accessory organs.

The alimentary canal is a Musculo-membranous tube, about thirty feet in length, extending from the mouth to the anus, and lined throughout its entire extent by mucuous membrane. At its commencement, which comprises the mouth, we find every provision for the mechanical division of the food (mastication), and for its admixture with a peculiar fluid secreted by the salivary glands (insalivation); beyond this is the pharynx and oesophagus, the organs of deglutition, which convey the food into that part of the alimentary canal (the stomach) in which the principal chemical changes occur; in the stomach, the reduction and solution of the food takes place; in the small intestines, the nutritive principles of the food (the chyle), by its admixture with the bile and pancreatic fluid, are separated from that portion which passes into the large intestine, and which is expelled from the system.

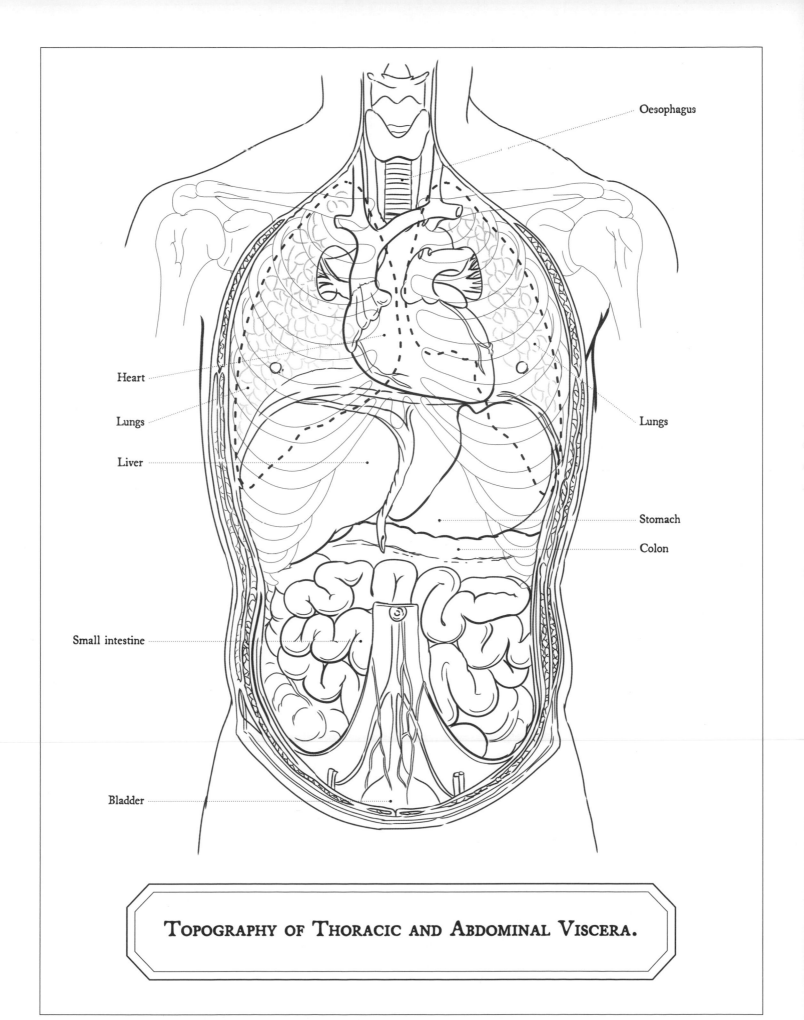

Oesophagus

Heart

Lungs

Lungs

Liver

Stomach

Colon

Small intestine

Bladder

TOPOGRAPHY OF THORACIC AND ABDOMINAL VISCERA.

The thorax is a conical, osseous framework, connected with the middle region of the spine. The viscera contained in the thorax are the great central organ of circulation, the heart, enclosed in its membranous bag, the pericardium; and the organs of respiration, the lungs, invested by the pleurae.

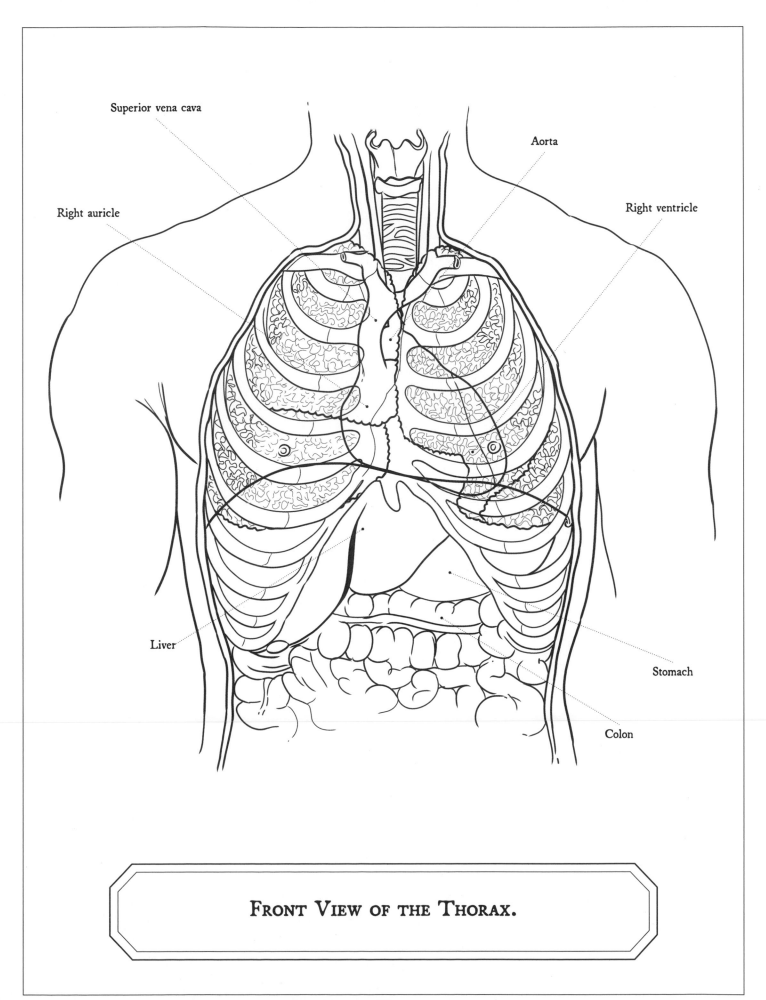

Superior vena cava

Aorta

Right auricle

Right ventricle

Liver

Stomach

Colon

FRONT VIEW OF THE THORAX.

The lungs are the essential organs of respiration; they are two in number, placed one in each of the lateral cavities of the chest, separated from each other by the heart and other contents of the mediastinum. Each lung is divided into two lobes, an upper and lower, by a long and deep fissure, which extends from the upper part of the posterior border of the organ, about three inches from its apex, downwards and forwards to the lower part of its anterior border. In the right lung the upper lobe is partially divided by a second and shorter fissure, which extends from the middle of the preceding, forwards and upwards, to the anterior margin of the organ, marking off a small triangular portion, the middle lobe.

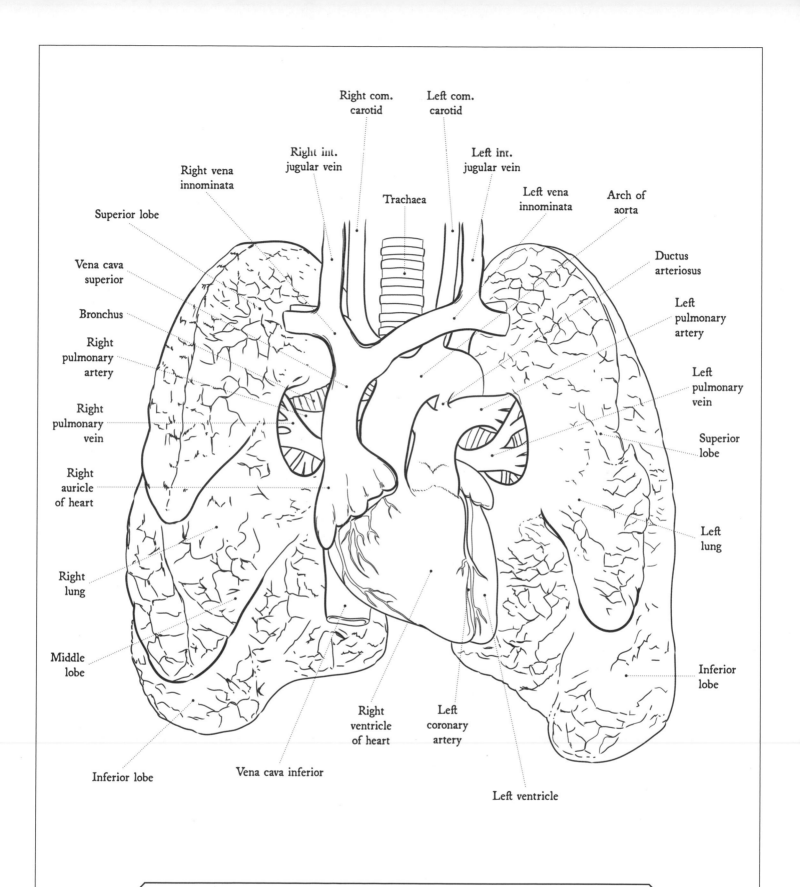

Right com. carotid

Left com. carotid

Right int. jugular vein

Left int. jugular vein

Right vena innominata

Trachaea

Left vena innominata

Arch of aorta

Superior lobe

Ductus arteriosus

Vena cava superior

Left pulmonary artery

Bronchus

Right pulmonary artery

Left pulmonary vein

Right pulmonary vein

Superior lobe

Right auricle of heart

Left lung

Right lung

Middle lobe

Inferior lobe

Inferior lobe

Vena cava inferior

Right ventricle of heart

Left coronary artery

Left ventricle

FRONT VIEW OF THE HEART AND LUNGS.

Each lung is invested, upon its external surface, by an
exceedingly delicate serous membrane, the pleura, which
encloses the organ as far as its root, and is then reflected
upon the inner surface of the thorax.
The portion of the serous membrane investing the surface
of the lung and dipping into the fissures between its lobes,
is called the pleura pulmonalis (visceral layer of pleura),
while that which lines the inner surface of the chest
is called the pleura costalis (parietal layer of pleura).
The space between these two layers is called the cavity
of the pleura, but it must be borne in mind that in the
healthy condition the two layers are in contact and there
is no real cavity, until the lung becomes collapsed and
a separation of it from the wall of the chest takes place.
Each pleura is therefore a shut sac, one occupying the
right, the other the left half of the thorax.

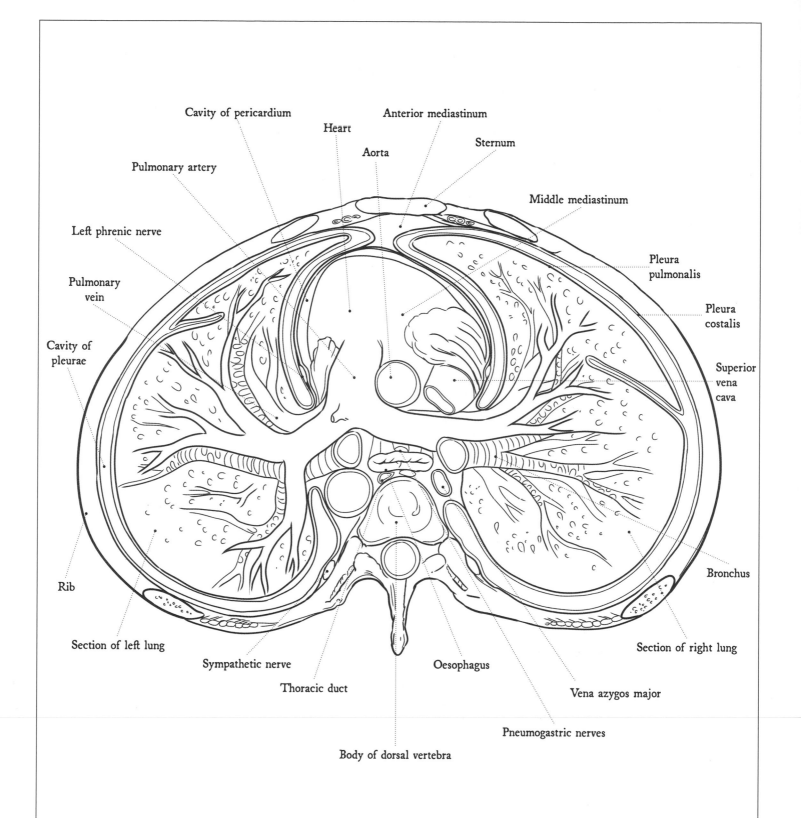

Cavity of pericardium

Heart

Anterior mediastinum

Aorta

Sternum

Pulmonary artery

Middle mediastinum

Left phrenic nerve

Pleura pulmonalis

Pulmonary vein

Pleura costalis

Cavity of pleurae

Superior vena cava

Rib

Bronchus

Section of left lung

Section of right lung

Sympathetic nerve

Oesophagus

Thoracic duct

Vena azygos major

Pneumogastric nerves

Body of dorsal vertebra

A TRANSVERSE SECTION OF THE THORAX, SHOWING THE RELATIVE POSITION OF THE VISCERA AND THE REFLECTIONS OF THE PLEURAE.

The aorta is the main trunk of a series of vessels, which,
arising from the heart, conveys the red oxygenated blood
to every part of the body for its nutrition. The vessel
commences at the upper part of the left ventricle, and
after ascending for a short distance, arches backwards
to the left side, over the root of the left lung, descends
within the thorax on the left side of the vertebral column,
passes through the aortic opening in the diaphragm, and
entering the abdominal cavity, terminates.

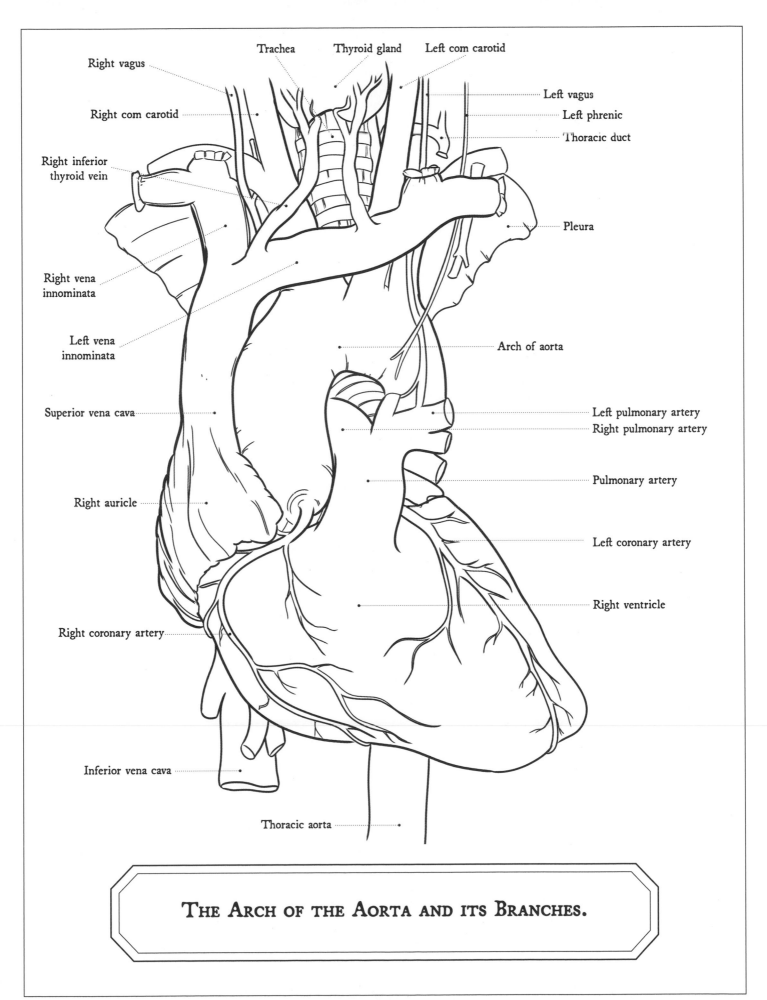

Right vagus

Trachea   Thyroid gland   Left com carotid

Right com carotid

Left vagus

Left phrenic

Thoracic duct

Right inferior
thyroid vein

Pleura

Right vena
innominata

Left vena
innominata

Arch of aorta

Superior vena cava

Left pulmonary artery

Right pulmonary artery

Pulmonary artery

Right auricle

Left coronary artery

Right ventricle

Right coronary artery

Inferior vena cava

Thoracic aorta

THE ARCH OF THE AORTA AND ITS BRANCHES.

The abdomen is the largest cavity of the trunk of the
body, and is separated, below, from the pelvic cavity by
the brim of the pelvis. This cavity contains the greater
part of the alimentary canal, some of the accessory
organs to digestion, the liver, pancreas and spleen, and
the kidneys and supra-renal capsules. Most of these
structures are covered by an extensive and complicated
serous membrane, the peritoneum. The abdomen is
artificially divided into certain regions. The middle region
of the upper zone is called the epigastric; and the two
lateral regions, the right and left hypochondriac.
The central region of the middle zone is the umbilical;
and the two lateral regions, the right and left lumbar.
The middle region of the lower zone is the hypogastric
or pubic region; and the lateral regions are the right and
left inguinal.

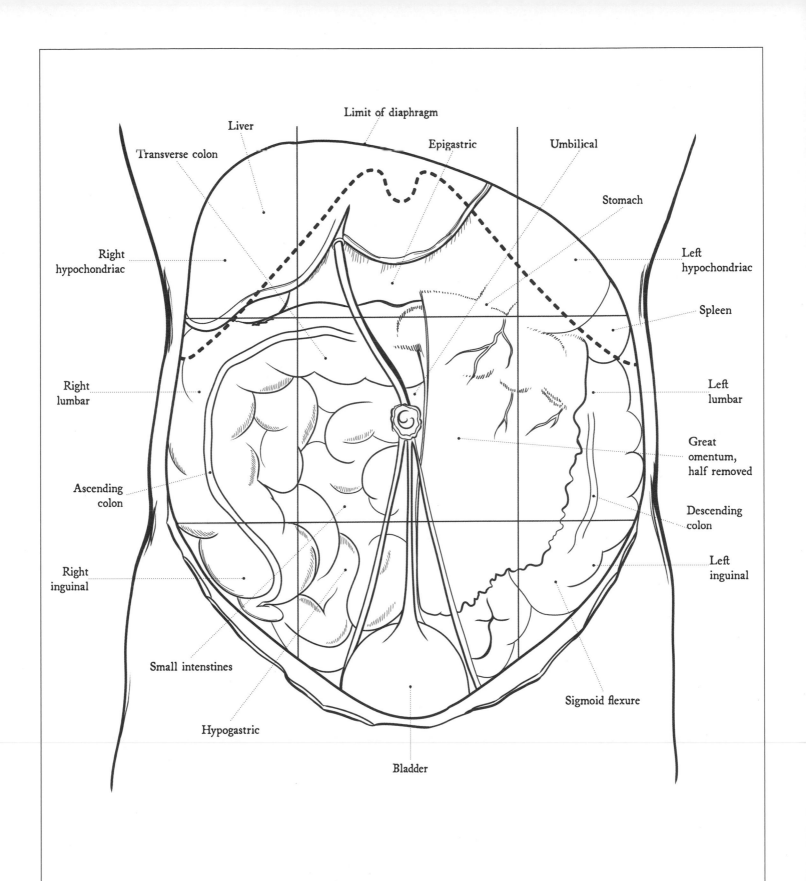

Limit of diaphragm

Liver

Transverse colon

Epigastric

Umbilical

Stomach

Right
hypochondriac

Left
hypochondriac

Spleen

Right
lumbar

Left
lumbar

Great
omentum,
half removed

Ascending
colon

Descending
colon

Right
inguinal

Left
inguinal

Small intenstines

Sigmoid flexure

Hypogastric

Bladder

THE REGIONS OF THE ABDOMEN AND THEIR CONTENTS.

The abdominal aorta commences at the aortic opening of
the diaphragm, and descending a little to the left side of
the vertebral column, terminates on the left side of the
body of the fourth lumbar vertebra, where it divides into
the two common iliac arteries.

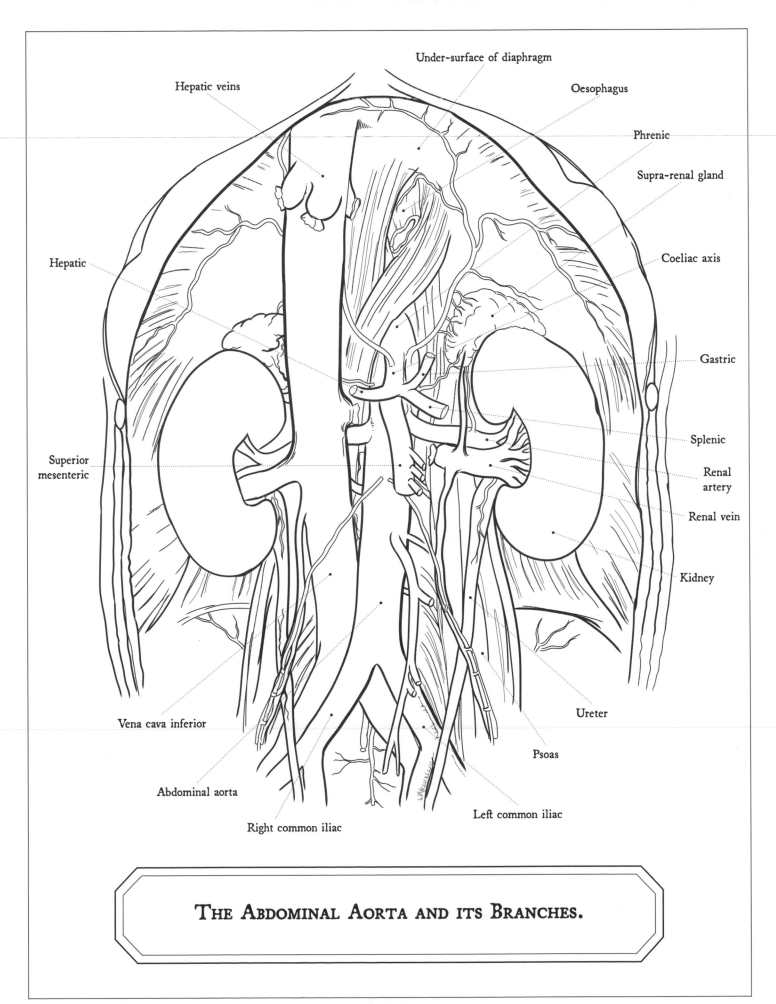

Under-surface of diaphragm

Hepatic veins

Oesophagus

Phrenic

Supra-renal gland

Hepatic

Coeliac axis

Gastric

Splenic

Superior
mesenteric

Renal
artery

Renal vein

Kidney

Ureter

Vena cava inferior

Psoas

Abdominal aorta

Left common iliac

Right common iliac

THE ABDOMINAL AORTA AND ITS BRANCHES.

The coeliac axis is a short thick trunk, about half an inch in length, arising from the aorta, and divides into three large branches, the gastric, hepatic and splenic occasionally giving off one of the phrenic arteries.

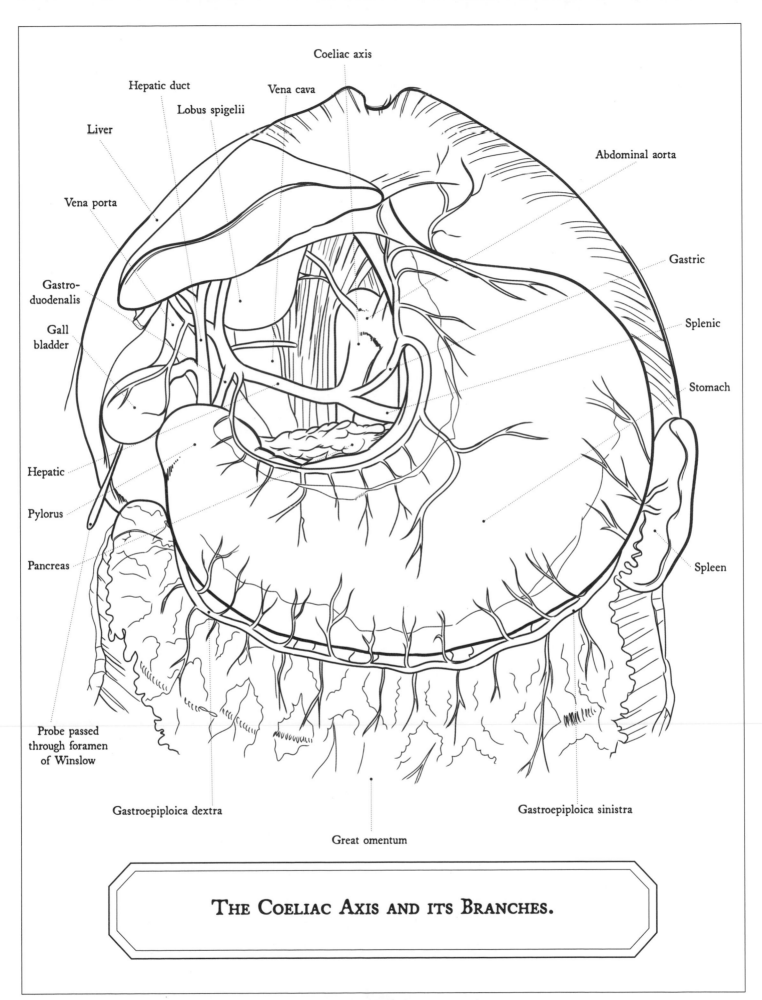

Coeliac axis

Hepatic duct

Lobus spigelii

Vena cava

Liver

Abdominal aorta

Vena porta

Gastric

Gastro-
duodenalis

Splenic

Gall
bladder

Stomach

Hepatic

Pylorus

Pancreas

Spleen

Probe passed
through foramen
of Winslow

Gastroepiploica dextra

Gastroepiploica sinistra

Great omentum

THE COELIAC AXIS AND ITS BRANCHES.

The liver is a glandular organ of large size, intended
mainly for the secretion of the bile, but effecting also
important changes in certain constituents of the blood in
their passage through the gland. It is situated in the right
hypochondriac region, and extends across the epigastrium
into the left hypochondrium. It is the largest gland in the
body, weighing from three to four pounds. It measures, in
its transverse diameter, from ten to twelve inches; from
six to seven in its antero-posterior; and is about three
inches thick at the back part of the right lobe, which is
the thickest part.

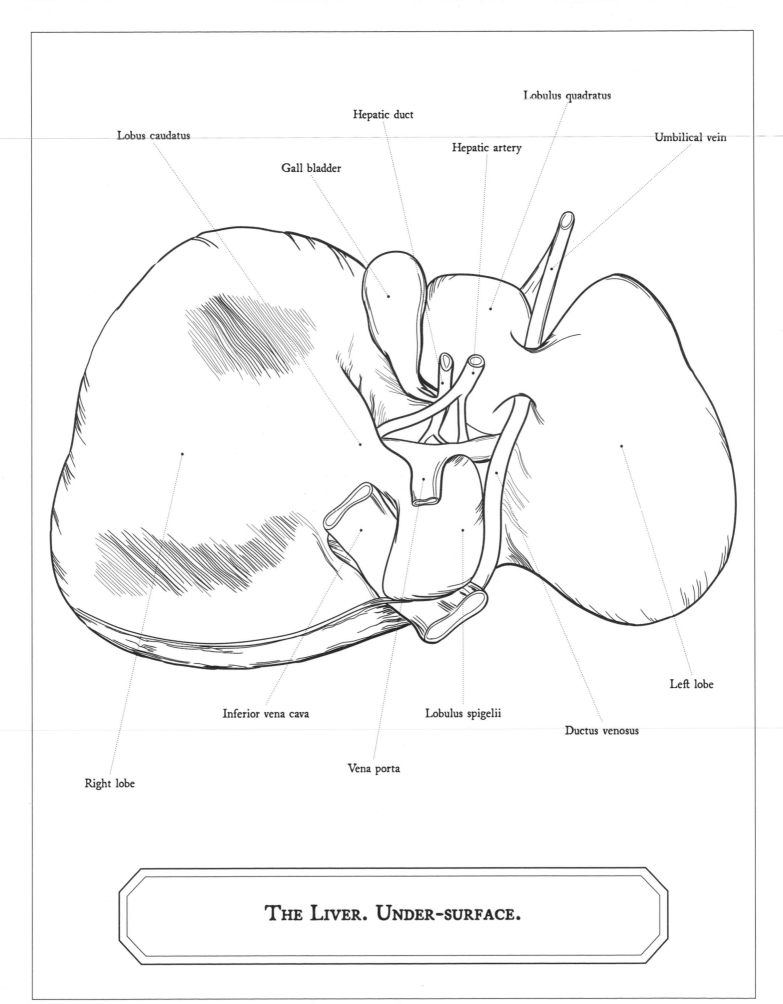

Lobulus quadratus

Hepatic duct

Hepatic artery

Umbilical vein

Lobus caudatus

Gall bladder

Right lobe

Inferior vena cava

Vena porta

Lobulus spigelii

Ductus venosus

Left lobe

The Liver. Under-surface.

The kidneys are two glandular organs, intended for the secretion of the urine. They are situated at the back part of the abdominal cavity, behind the peritoneum. They are usually surrounded by a considerable quantity of fat, and are retained in their position by the vessels which pass to and from them. The cortical substance forms about three-fourths of the gland. It is soft, reddish, granular, easily lacerated and contains numerous small, red bodies disseminated through it in every part. The medullary substance consists of pale, reddish conical masses, the pyramids of Malpighi.

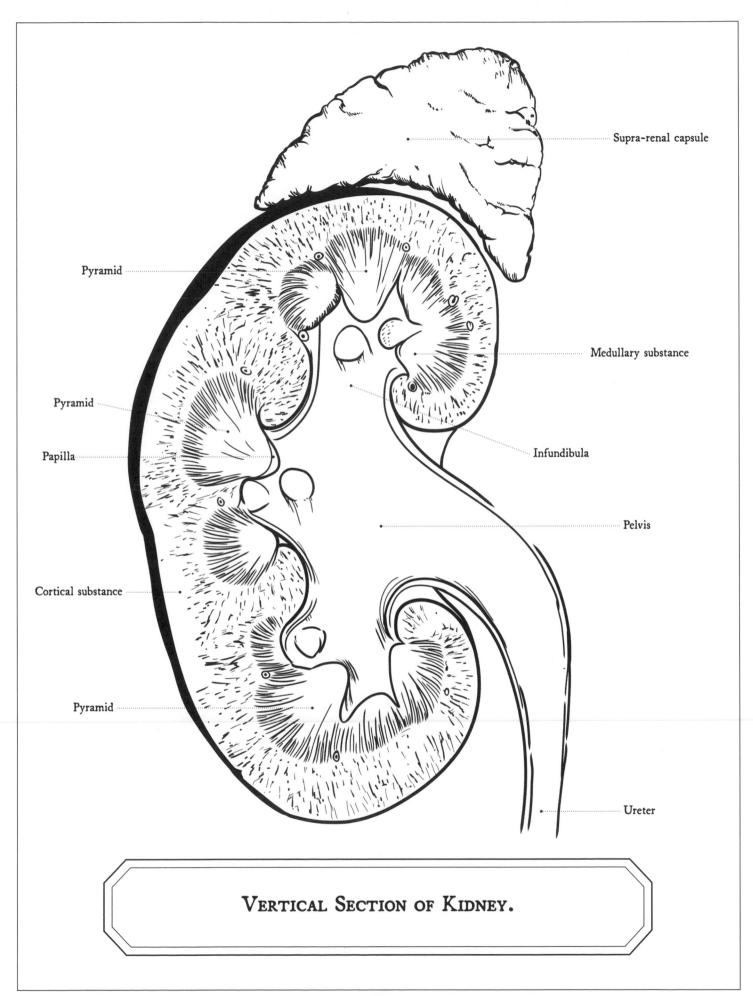

Supra-renal capsule

Pyramid

Medullary substance

Pyramid

Infundibula

Papilla

Pelvis

Cortical substance

Pyramid

Ureter

VERTICAL SECTION OF KIDNEY.

The pancreas is a conglomerate gland. It is situated
transversely across the posterior wall of the abdomen.
Its length varies from six to eight inches, its breadth is
an inch and a half, and its thickness from half an inch
to an inch, being thicker at its right extremity and along
its upper border. Its weight varies from two to three and
a half ounces, but it may reach six ounces. In structure,
the pancreas closely resembles the salivary glands; but it
is looser and softer in its texture.

The spleen is usually classified together with the thyroid,
supra-renal glands and thymus, as one of the ductless
glands. It is of an oblong flattened form, soft, of very
brittle consistence, highly vascular, of a dark bluish-red,
and situated in the left hypochondriac region, embracing
the cardiac end of the stomach.

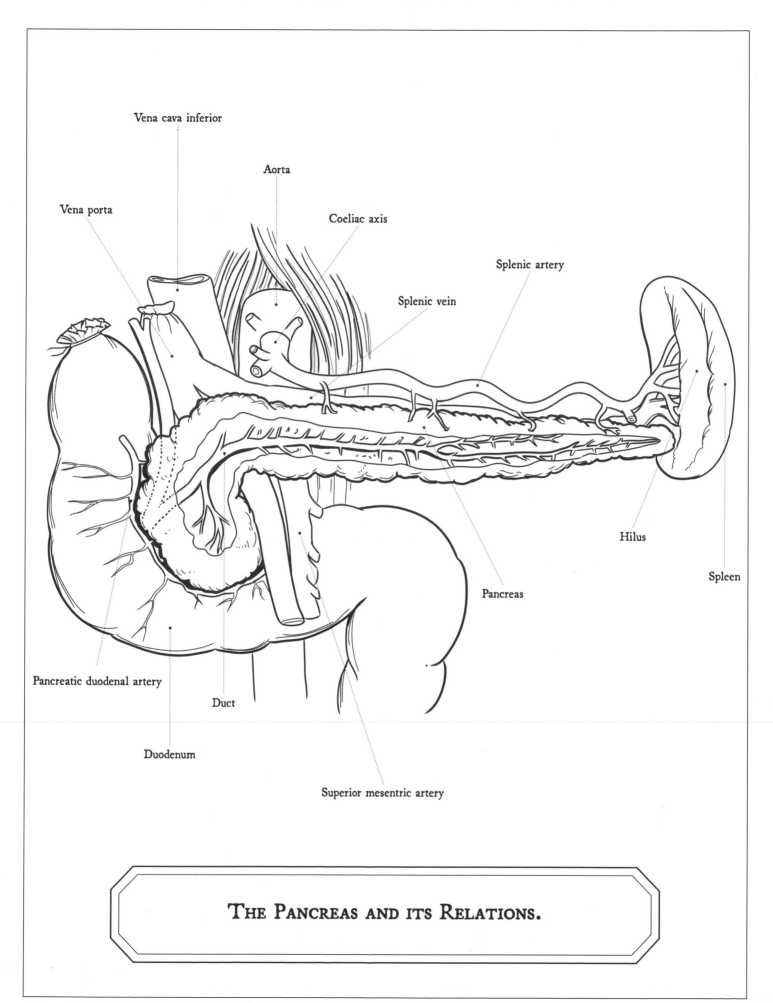

Vena cava inferior

Aorta

Vena porta

Coeliac axis

Splenic artery

Splenic vein

Hilus

Spleen

Pancreas

Pancreatic duodenal artery

Duct

Duodenum

Superior mesentric artery

THE PANCREAS AND ITS RELATIONS.

In the neck, the two common carotids resemble each other closely. Starting from each side, each vessel passes obliquely upwards, from behind the sterno-clavicular articulation, to a level with the upper border of the thyroid cartilage, where it divides into the external and internal carotid. The common carotid artery is contained in a sheath, derived from the deep cervical fascia, which also encloses the internal jugular vein and pneumogastric nerve, the vein, lying on the outer side of the artery, and the nerve between the artery and vein, on a plane posterior to both.

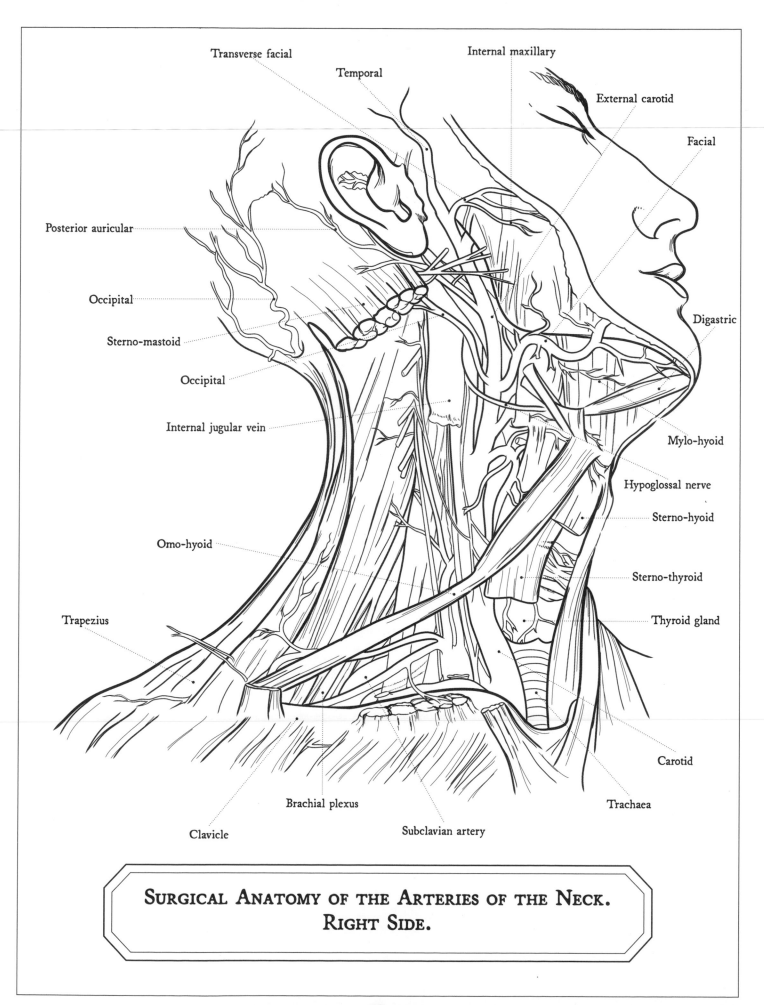

Transverse facial

Temporal

Internal maxillary

External carotid

Facial

Posterior auricular

Occipital

Sterno-mastoid

Occipital

Internal jugular vein

Omo-hyoid

Trapezius

Digastric

Mylo-hyoid

Hypoglossal nerve

Sterno-hyoid

Sterno-thyroid

Thyroid gland

Carotid

Trachaea

Clavicle

Brachial plexus

Subclavian artery

SURGICAL ANATOMY OF THE ARTERIES OF THE NECK.
RIGHT SIDE.

These may be divided into three groups: the veins of the
exterior of the head, the veins of the neck and the veins
of the diploë and interior of the cranium. The veins of
the exterior of the heard are:

Facial.
Temporal.
Internal maxillary.
Temporo-maxillary.
Posterior auricular.
Occipital.

The veins of the neck, which return the blood from the
head and face, are:

External jugular.
Anterior jugular.
Posterior external jugular.
Internal jugular.
Vertebral.

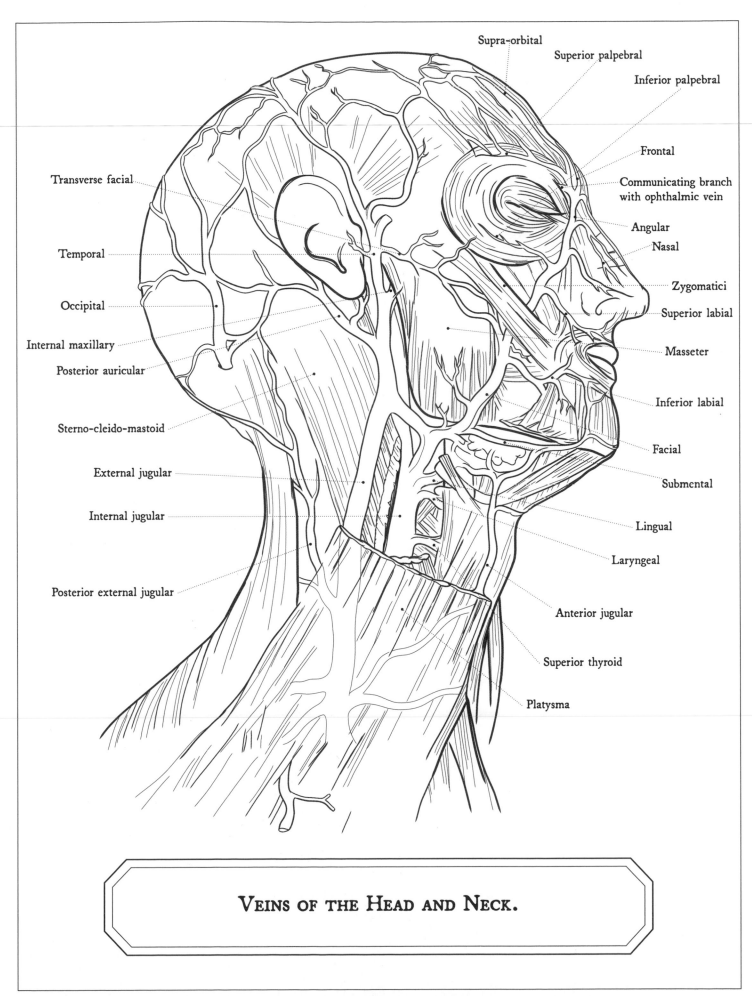

Supra-orbital

Superior palpebral

Inferior palpebral

Frontal

Communicating branch
with ophthalmic vein

Angular

Nasal

Zygomatici

Superior labial

Masseter

Inferior labial

Facial

Submental

Lingual

Laryngeal

Anterior jugular

Superior thyroid

Platysma

Transverse facial

Temporal

Occipital

Internal maxillary

Posterior auricular

Sterno-cleido-mastoid

External jugular

Internal jugular

Posterior external jugular

VEINS OF THE HEAD AND NECK.

81

The ulnar artery, the larger of the two sub-divisions
of the brachial, commences a little below the bend
of the elbow, and crosses the inner side of the fore-
arm obliquely to the commencement of its lower half.
The radial artery appears, from its direction, to be the
continuation of the brachial, but, in size, it is smaller
than the ulnar.

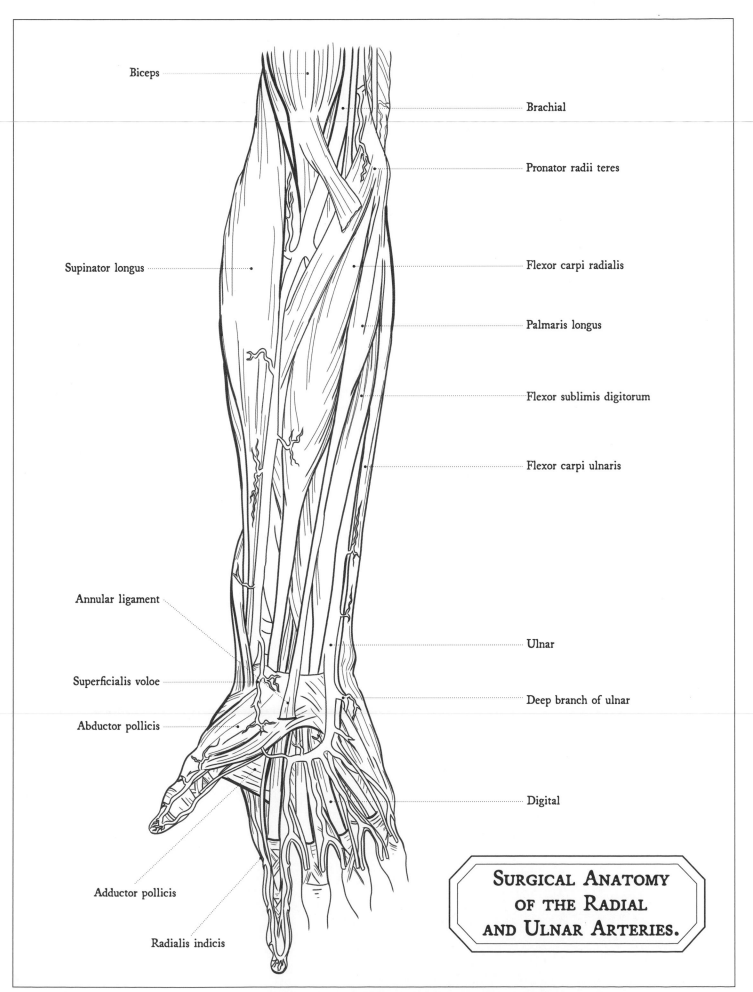

Biceps

Brachial

Pronator radii teres

Supinator longus

Flexor carpi radialis

Palmaris longus

Flexor sublimis digitorum

Flexor carpi ulnaris

Annular ligament

Superficialis voloe

Ulnar

Abductor pollicis

Deep branch of ulnar

Digital

Adductor pollicis

Radialis indicis

SURGICAL ANATOMY
OF THE RADIAL
AND ULNAR ARTERIES.

The axilla is a conical space, situated between the upper and lateral parts of the chest and inner side of the arm. The axillary artery and vein, with the brachial plexus of nerves, extend obliquely along the outer boundary of the axillary space, from its apex to its base, and are placed much nearer the anterior than the posterior wall, the vein lying to the inner or thoracic side of the artery, and altogether concealing it. The student should attentively consider the relation of the vessels and nerves in the several parts of the axilla; for it not unfrequently happens that the surgeon is called upon to extirpate diseased glands, or to remove a tumour from this situation. In performing such an operation, it will be necessary to proceed with much caution in the direction of the outer wall and apex of the space, as here the axillary vessels will be in danger of being wounded.

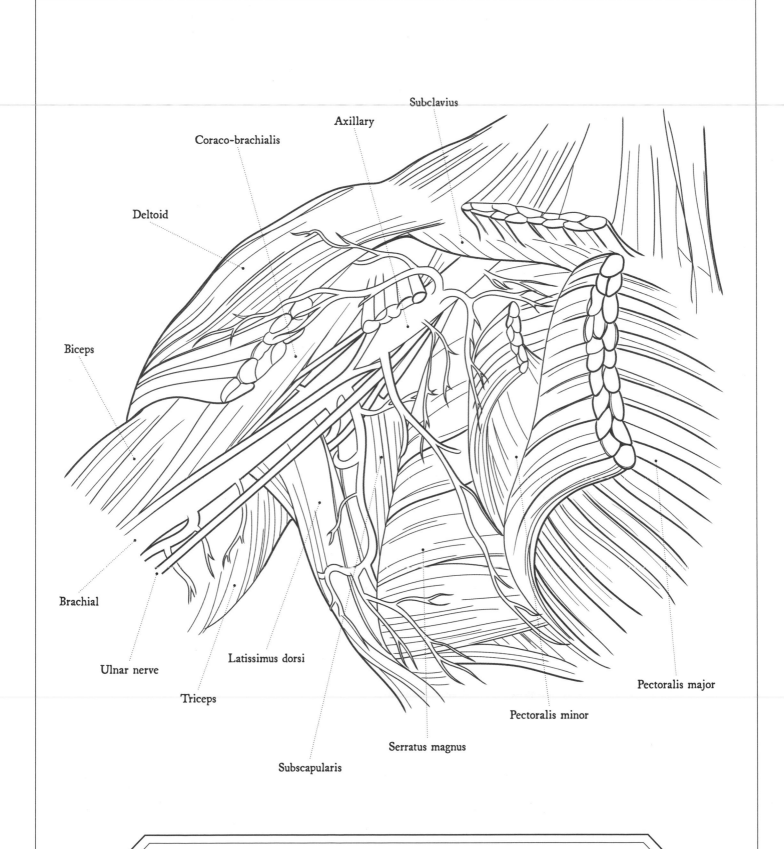

Subclavius

Axillary

Coraco-brachialis

Deltoid

Biceps

Brachial

Ulnar nerve

Triceps

Latissimus dorsi

Subscapularis

Serratus magnus

Pectoralis minor

Pectoralis major

SURGICAL ANATOMY OF THE AXILLARY ARTERY.

The portal venous system is composed of four large veins, which collect the venous blood from the viscera of digestion. The trunk formed by their union (vena portae) enters the liver, ramifies throughout its substance, and its branches again emerging from that organ as the hepatic veins terminate in the inferior vena cava. The veins forming the portal system are the inferior mesenteric, superior mesenteric, splenic and gastric.

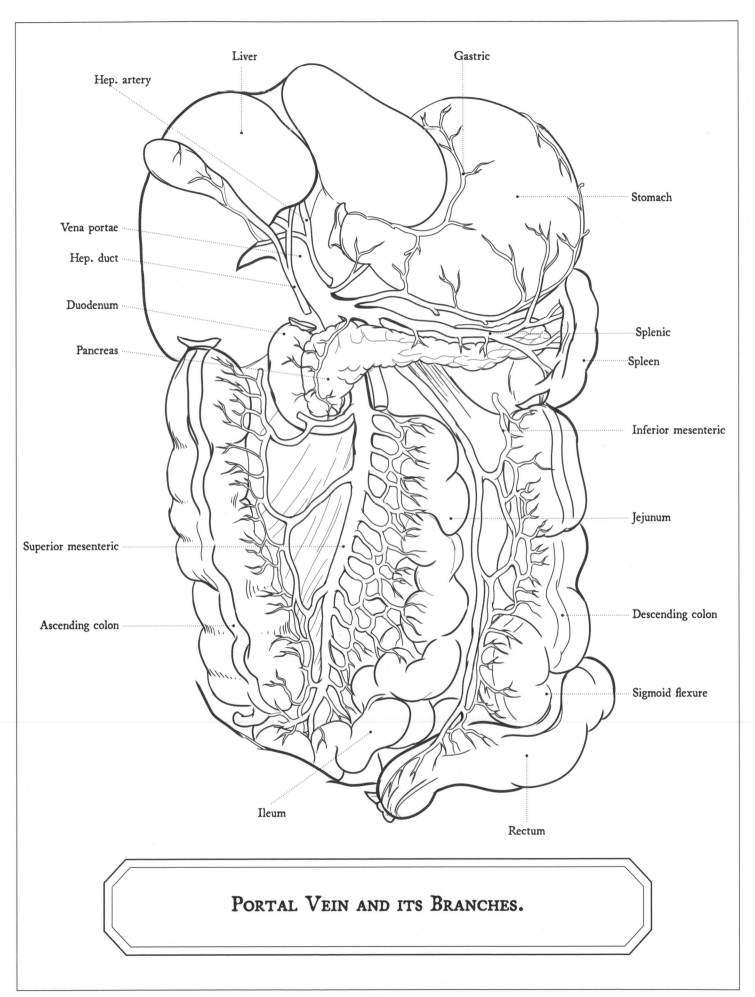

Hep. artery

Liver

Gastric

Vena portae

Hep. duct

Duodenum

Pancreas

Stomach

Splenic

Spleen

Superior mesenteric

Inferior mesenteric

Jejunum

Ascending colon

Descending colon

Sigmoid flexure

Ileum

Rectum

PORTAL VEIN AND ITS BRANCHES.

The brain (encephalon) is that portion of the cerebro-spinal axis that is contained in the cranial cavity. It is divided into four principal parts: viz. the cerebrum, the cerebellum, the pons Varolii and medulla oblongata.

The average weight of the brain in the adult male is 49 ½ oz, or a little more than 3 lb; that of the female, 44 oz. It appears that the weight of the brain increases rapidly up to the seventh year, more slowly to between sixteen and twenty, and still more slowly to between thirty and forty, when it reaches its maximum. Beyond this period, as age advances and the mental faculties decline, the brain diminishes slowly in weight.

The cerebrum, in man, constitutes the largest portion of the encephalon. Its upper surface is of an ovoidal form, broader behind than in front, convex in its general outline, and divided into two lateral halves or hemispheres, right and left, by the great longitudinal fissure.

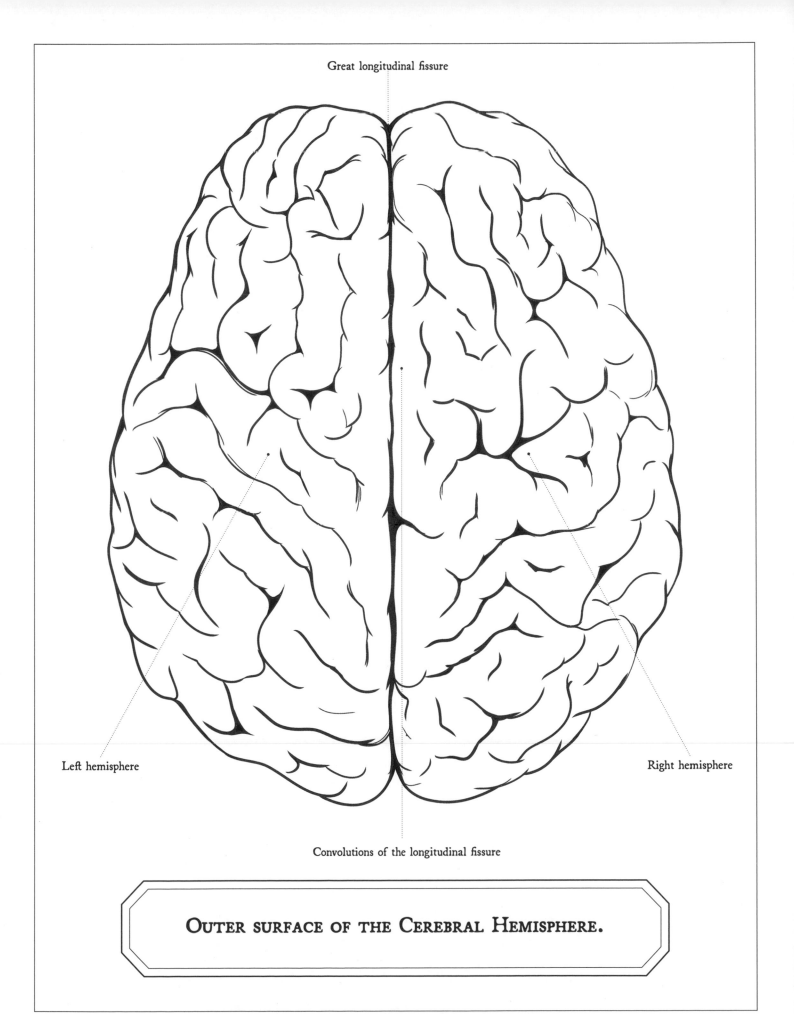

Great longitudinal fissure

Left hemisphere

Right hemisphere

Convolutions of the longitudinal fissure

OUTER SURFACE OF THE CEREBRAL HEMISPHERE.

The sympathetic nerve is so called from the opinion entertained that through it is produced a sympathy between the affections of distant organs. It consists of a series of ganglia, connected together by intervening cords, extending on each side of the vertebral column from the base of the skull to the coccyx.

The sympathetic nerve may be divided into several parts, and the number of ganglia of which each part is composed, may be thus arranged:

Cephalic portion	4 ganglia
Cervical	3 ganglia
Dorsal	12 ganglia
Lumbar	4 ganglia
Sacral	5 ganglia
Coccygeal	1 ganglion

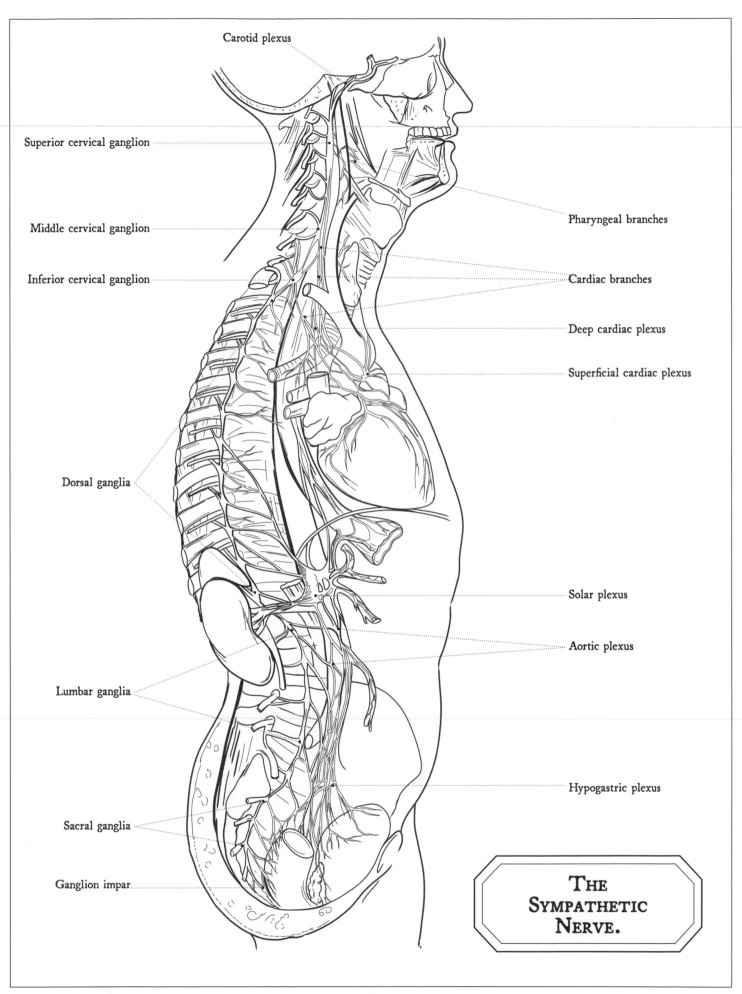

Carotid plexus

Superior cervical ganglion

Middle cervical ganglion

Inferior cervical ganglion

Dorsal ganglia

Lumbar ganglia

Sacral ganglia

Ganglion impar

Pharyngeal branches

Cardiac branches

Deep cardiac plexus

Superficial cardiac plexus

Solar plexus

Aortic plexus

Hypogastric plexus

THE
SYMPATHETIC
NERVE.

The mouth is placed at the commencement of the
alimentary canal; it is a nearly oval-shaped cavity,
in which the mastication of the food takes place. It is
bounded, in front, by the lips; laterally, by the lips;
laterally, by the cheeks and alveolar process of the upper
and lower jaw; above, by the hard palate and teeth of the
upper jaw; below, by the tongue, the mucous membrane
stretched between the under-surface of this organ and the
inner surface of the jaws, and by the teeth of the lower
jaw; behind by the soft palate and fauces. The lips are
two fleshy folds, which surround the orifice of the mouth,
formed externally of integument, internally of mucous
membrane. The palate forms the roof of the mouth; it
consists of two portions, the hard palate in front, the soft
palate behind. The cheeks form the side of the face, and
are continuous in front with the lips. The pharynx is that
part of the alimentary canal which is placed behind the
nose, mouth and larynx. It is a musculo-membranous sac,
somewhat conical in form.

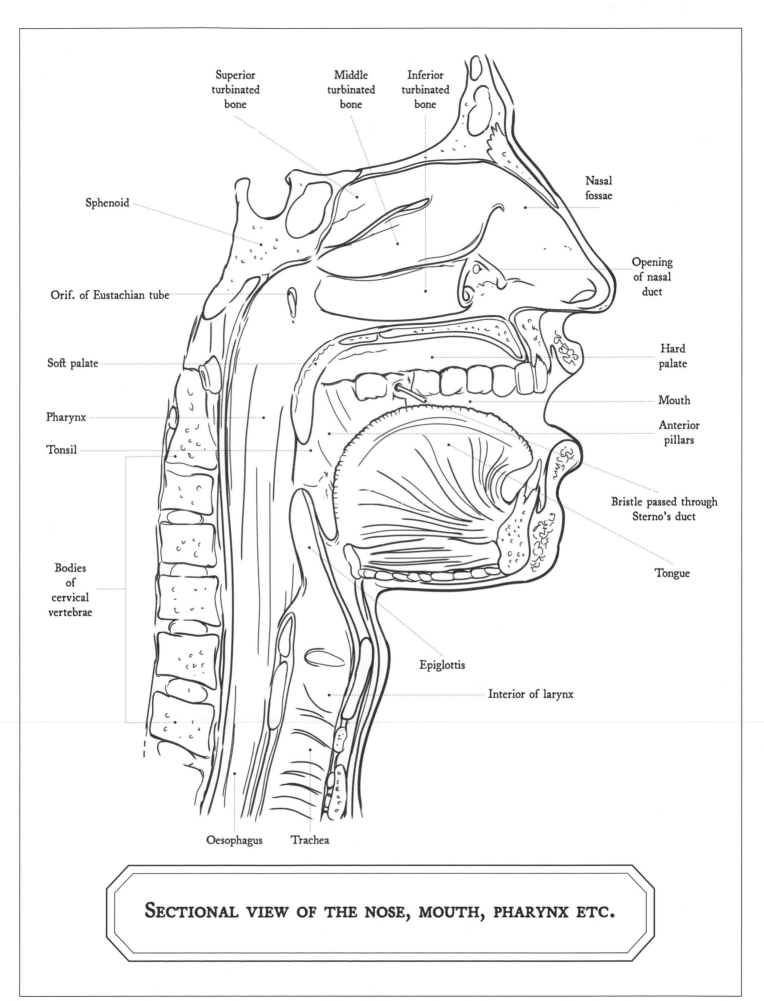

Superior turbinated bone

Middle turbinated bone

Inferior turbinated bone

Nasal fossae

Sphenoid

Opening of nasal duct

Orif. of Eustachian tube

Hard palate

Soft palate

Mouth

Pharynx

Anterior pillars

Tonsil

Bristle passed through Sterno's duct

Bodies of cervical vertebrae

Tongue

Epiglottis

Interior of larynx

Oesophagus

Trachea

SECTIONAL VIEW OF THE NOSE, MOUTH, PHARYNX ETC.

The organ of hearing consists of three parts: the external
ear, the middle ear or tympanum and the internal ear
or labyrinth. The external ear consists of an expanded
portion named pinna, or auricle, and the auditory canal
or meatus. The former serves to collect the vibrations
of the air constituting sound, and the latter conducts
those vibrations to the tympanum. The middle ear, or
tympanum, is an irregular cavity. It is filled with air, and
communicates with the pharynx by the Eustachian tube.
The tympanum is traversed by a chain of moveable bones,
which connect the membrana tympani with the labyrinth,
and serve to convey the vibrations communicated to the
membrana tympani across the cavity of the tympanum to
the internal ear. The internal ear is the essential part of
the acoustic organ, receiving the ultimate distribution of
the auditory nerve. It is called the labyrinth, from the
complexity of its communications, and consists of three
parts: the vestibule, semi-circular canals and choclea.
It comprises a series of cavities, channelled out of the
substance of the petrous bone, communicating externally
with the cavity of the tympanum; and internally, with
the meatus auditorius internus, which contains the
auditory nerve.

Mastoid cells

Semicircular canals

Incus

Vestibule

Malleus

Stapes

Cochlea

Tensor tympani

Eustachian tube

Meatus auditorius externus

Osseous portion

Pinna

Membrana tympani

Parotid gland

Cavity of tympanum

Cartilaginous portion

FRONT VIEW OF THE ORGAN OF HEARING. RIGHT SIDE.

LIST OF ILLUSTRATIONS

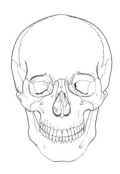